THE
SWIM
PRESCRIPTION

THE
SWIM
PRESCRIPTION

How Swimming Can Improve Your
Mood, Restore Health, Increase Physical
Fitness and Revitalize Your Life

ALEXANDER HUTCHISON, PHD

Hatherleigh Press is committed to preserving and protecting the natural resources of the earth. Environmentally responsible and sustainable practices are embraced within the company's mission statement.

Visit us at www.hatherleighpress.com and register online for free offers, discounts, special events, and more.

THE SWIM PRESCRIPTION

Library of Congress Cataloging-in-Publication Data is available upon request.
ISBN 978-157826-846-7

All Hatherleigh Press titles are available for bulk purchase, special promotions, and premiums. For information about reselling and special purchase opportunities, please call 1-800-528-2550 and ask for the Special Sales Manager.

Cover and Interior Design by Carolyn Kasper

10 9 8 7 6 5 4 3 2 1
Printed in the United States

For Charles van der Horst

"Dr. Charlie"

Contents

Why Swim? How Swimming Became My Prescription   ix

PART 1:
SWIMMING AS PRESCRIPTION

1. Swimming For Your Health   3

2. Swimming and Cardiovascular Health   17

3. Swimming and Pulmonary Health   31

4. Swimming and Bone Health   45

5. Swimming for Weight Loss and Weight Management   51

6. Swimming as a Treatment for Neurological Disorders   59

7. Swimming for Pain Management   69

8. Swimming for Mental Health and Wellness   73

PART 2:
SWIMMING AS A LIFESTYLE

9. Getting Started   83

10. Learning the Basics   89

11. Swimming Equipment: The Ins and Outs   99

12. Swimming Technique 101   107

PART 3:
PRACTICAL APPLICATIONS & NEXT STEPS

13. Basic Nutrition for Swimming Performance   129

14. Strength Training for Swimmers   137

15. Cross Training & Open Water Swimming   141

PART 4:
SWIM PRESCRIPTION WORKOUTS

12-Week Program: Level I   *150*

12-Week Program: Level II   *167*

12-Week Program: Level III   *184*

Afterword   *201*

Acknowledgments   *205*

Reference Tables   *207*

About the Author   *231*

References   *233*

Why Swim?
How Swimming Became My Prescription

The first sport that I excelled in was swimming.

Introduced to the water as an infant, my mother has a collection of faded pictures from the mid-70s of me splashing around in our apartment complex's pool in Staten Island. At the age of three, we moved to Brownsville Texas, and most of my swimming shifted from pools to the shores of the Gulf coast.

After my parents divorced when I was eight, I went through a period of depression and anxiety. I lost my appetite, leading to a period of rapid weight loss. I felt lonely and isolated and began expressing myself with my fists rather than my words. My preferred activity became picking fights with the biggest bullies I could find—not exactly a surefire path to success or happiness.

Frustrated and concerned, my mother decided that she would try to channel my aggression into something more constructive: sports. We tried soccer, but I didn't have the ball skills to play in the field, and although I was a pretty good goalie, that position only served to bring out my more aggressive tendencies—exactly the opposite of the intended result. Goalies aren't supposed to get red cards, after all.

Over my first five games, I earned three of them.

At the suggestion of a family friend, my mother took me to the Blue Dolphins Swim Team for a tryout. We arrived near the end of the practice session; the six-lane pool was packed with swimmers of all ages, both boys and girls. After completing my tryout (which consisted of successfully swimming across the length of the 25-yard pool without drowning), my coach asked if I wanted to join in for "sprint time." I nodded my head in the affirmative, as the first wave of high school boys got up on the blocks. They took to their marks, the coach barked a loud "HUP!", and they *exploded* off the blocks, hitting the water with a stealthy "shoo" and rumbling down the pool.

My coach, a man by the name of Ruben, asked if I was ready. The boys in the next wave looked to be in middle school, but they were still pretty imposing. I didn't even answer, too busy running to the outside lane, and climbing onto the diving block. No goggles on, cut-off jeans with tendrils of denim hanging down my spindly thighs. My mother told Ruben, loud enough for everyone to hear, that I hadn't yet learned to dive and that I probably shouldn't use the block, maybe start from the deck, or worse still, from a push, already in the water.

You know that feeling when your mom licks her fingers and then uses those slimy digits to clean a speck of food off your face in front of all of your friends?

Yeah, exactly.

"*Mom!* I can do it!"

Fast forward five years, I was a high school freshman on a new club swim team in Houston, Texas. After three very successful summers on the University of Houston summer league swim team, a brief, pre-internet search for a new club led us to a coach with a reputation for having a big, successful team. He was a wonderful person, and he certainly had produced many very accomplished swimmers. But I distinctly remember being told before my first practice that he "didn't believe in sprinting." His philosophy centered on hours of long distance, moderately paced swimming. By the end of that year, I was actually swimming slower in my favorite events. Two to three hours a day in an outdoor pool, in the winter, was not fun. It was cold and boring. I decided to quit, but I was obligated to swim in one more meet that season.

During our warm-up session for the meet, I saw all the teams doing the same, old, unmotivated routine. 500 swim, 200 kick, 200 pull, two dive starts, go sit on your towel with your juice box and Fruit Roll-up, and wait to swim your first event without a chance to warm-up or cool-down between races. But there was one small team of 10 or 11 kids who were doing something very different. Three girls were in the water, swimming with what looked like big bungee cords wrapped around their waists. On the other end of these long elastic bands were three teammates standing on the deck. The three girls in the water swam against the resistance to other end of the pool. With one hand firmly gripping the wall, they rotated the belts around so that the cord attachment was in front of their waists.

I was completely enthralled. "What the hell is this?" I said to myself. The big bungee cords were stretched out to 25 yards and vibrating menacingly as though they would snap at any moment. At the call of, "GO!" all three girls took off, arms and legs churning up a huge wake behind them. At the same time, their three teammates holding the other ends of the cords started frantically reeling them in so that there was no slack, and the elastic recoil of the cord would be maintained for the whole length of the sprint. These girls were freaking fast! Never a shy person, I was on my feet and walking fast to introduce myself to their coach. I asked her if I could give it a try. She agreed, and I joined my new team that day.

This was my first introduction to the versatility of swimming not just as a sport, but as a way of life.

Swimming as an exercise modality imparts unique benefits to the cardiovascular, respiratory, musculoskeletal, and metabolic systems, and our emotional health, that other land-based physical activities do not. So, what's the difference? After all, exercise is exercise. Well, it all comes down to H_2O. Being in an aquatic environment changes our entire internal milieu, "resetting" our bodies, if you will, to a healthier homeostatic balance than we experience when participating in land-based exercises. This is true for all ages, but particularly for the youngest and oldest among us.

THIS BOOK

My purpose in writing this book is to make the case for why swimming is an activity not just for health, but for life. The book is divided into four sections:

Part 1: Swimming as Prescription

In this first section, I go in-depth on all of the health benefits that swimming provides, in many instances surpassing what can be accomplished with running or cycling. Each topic includes a thorough explanation of how each organ system works and how swimming benefits you, all presented in an easy-to-understand way without technical jargon.

Part 2: Swimming as a Lifestyle

In this section, I discuss the practical application of the science behind swimming. For example:

- What equipment you need to get started
- A detailed description of each of the four primary strokes
- How to determine your swimming paces for recovery, fitness maintenance, and improving your speed.

Reading this section prepares you to get the best start possible for your swimming regimen.

Part 3: Practical Applications and Next Steps

Here, I cover some of the connected elements that you will need to complement your new life as a swimmer, including:

- Basic nutrition for a healthy, happy life
- Strength training for swimmers
- How to safely add open water swimming into your routine

Swim Prescription Workouts

In this section, I've provided detailed 12-week training plans for beginner, intermediate, and advanced swimmers, categorized as Levels I–III. This section also includes some simple instructions on how to construct your own training plans; i.e., how many days per week, how many sets, what pace, what stroke, etc.

It is my hope that, by the time you've finished reading this book you will be not only prepared, but *excited*, to enter the exhilarating world of swimming as lifestyle.

PART 1

SWIMMING AS PRESCRIPTION

CHAPTER 1

Swimming For Your Health

I t is a safe bet that your primary motivation for learning how to swim is to help you get in shape, burn fat and lose weight. In other words, you want to improve your physical fitness. That's a wonderful goal, and swimming is a perfect activity for anyone looking to make healthy lifestyle changes by including exercise into their routine.

But before you stick one toe in the water, it's best to learn as much as you can about what we're really talking about when we say we want to be in "better shape." It's one thing to look good In a swimsuit, but what does it really mean to be physically fit?

PHYSICAL FITNESS: JUST THE FACTS

There are several popular (and often complex) definitions of what it means to be physically fit. In its simplest form, physical fitness is the body's ability to deliver oxygen (O_2) and fuel—in the form of both carbs (glucose) and fat—to the muscles. When these ingredients are present in the muscle cells, they are fed into a series of chemical reactions that produce a very important substance called adenosine triphosphate, or ATP. The production and use of ATP are what we collectively refer to as our **metabolism**—that term you hear about all the time when discussing a new diet or health trend. Our metabolism plays a big part in how exercise impacts our body, and ATP plays a big part in how our metabolism functions.

ATP

ATP is the energy unit for life, used to drive all the reactions that keep us alive. A few examples include providing the energy for muscle contractions, heart beats, and keeping our electrolyte levels in balance so that our nervous system can function properly. Interestingly, as important as ATP is to life, we keep very little in reserve. If you stopped your production of ATP right now while reading this sentence, you would be dead before you finished the paragraph. It is estimated that we have between 2–5 seconds worth of ATP in reserve at any given time. This means that we must constantly deliver the raw materials of O_2, glucose, and fat to our tissues, and remove the metabolic waste products that are produced, namely carbon dioxide (CO_2).

We have evolved to metabolize glucose both with and without O_2. Energy pathways that can work without O_2 are termed **anaerobic**, while those that require O_2 are **aerobic**. The complete metabolism of one molecule of glucose produces 32 ATP and requires both the anaerobic and aerobic pathways to work together like an assembly line. The process of glucose metabolism begins with the anaerobic pathway called glycolysis, which literally translates to sugar = glyco, splitting = lysis. The products of glycolysis feed into the aerobic pathways. When we need to produce ATP very quickly, as we do when engaged in high-intensity exercise, glycolysis speeds up dramatically.

There are two drawbacks to this approach, however:

- Glycolysis alone is very inefficient, only producing 2 ATP per glucose (the other 30 ATP are made by our aerobic pathways).

- More importantly, as glycolysis speeds up to meet ATP demand during high-intensity exercise, it makes more products than can be handled by the aerobic pathways. In other words, the assembly line gets backed up. This leads to the buildup of lactic acid. This is the stuff that makes your muscles burn and causes fatigue.

The fact that we *can* make ATP in the absence of O_2 does not mean that these conditions exist in our muscles during high-intensity exercise. To be clear, the amount of O_2 present in the muscles never drops below the critical threshold required to run our aerobic pathways; we just don't deliver enough O_2 to the muscles to run our aerobic pathways any faster, so we have to turn to glycolysis to make up the difference. Think about the activities that you do when you "feel the burn." These are short duration, explosive, very high-intensity bouts that last from 10–90 seconds at most. You then require a lot of active recovery before you can repeat another bout. This is quite different from going for a long, sustained jog with a friend and chatting with them the whole time. Under these more "aerobic" conditions, you're delivering plenty enough O_2 to the muscles to allow your aerobic pathways to make enough ATP to keep you running comfortably for an hour or more.

FAT

Now, let's switch gears and talk about our other fuel source, fat. Unlike glucose, which requires both glycolysis and our aerobic pathways to be completely metabolized, fat can only be metabolized aerobically. When we refer to "fat" in the nutritional sense, we are talking about a family of molecules called fatty acids. Whereas glucose has a fixed size, the length of fatty acids varies from short, to medium, and long-chain fatty acids. This means that fat as a general term does not translate to a set amount of ATP, unlike glucose (32 ATP). But, on average, metabolism of one gram of fat generates 2.25 times more energy than one gram of glucose.

So, the obvious question is, why do we bother burning glucose when fat provides so much more energy? Although we have effectively limitless supplies of stored fat, we can only store between 2–4 hours' worth of glucose in our liver and muscles. The tradeoff is speed of combustion. The mantra in exercise nutrition is that "Carbs burn faster than fats!" At rest, and during low-intensity exercise, we preferentially burn fat because it packs so much more of an ATP punch than does glucose. But as exercise intensity increases, we switch to using glucose because it can be metabolized to make ATP faster.

It is precisely this balance in the amounts of glucose and fat that we burn that defines our fitness level. In short, aerobic fitness really means how long you can delay fatigue during continuous, moderate to high-intensity exercise. Let me explain how this works. Glycolysis takes place in the liquid interior of our cells, an area called the cytoplasm. Aerobic endurance training has little impact on the number of glycolytic enzymes present in the cytoplasm. By contrast, the aerobic pathways are housed in complex structures called mitochondria, often referred to as the "powerhouses" of our cells. Think of the mitochondria as furnaces that generate ATP when we feed them glucose and fat to burn in the presence of O_2. Endurance training leads to significant increases in the number, and size, of the mitochondria present in our muscle cells. The more furnaces we have, the more fat we can burn at higher intensities of exercise. If we shift to burning more fat, we will burn less glucose.

This delays the onset of fatigue in two ways:

- We burn through our stored glucose (called glycogen) slower. Running out of muscle glycogen is like having your hybrid car run out of gas, the car can still roll, but you're going to have to use the battery instead, and the top speed of the car is much slower while using the battery. When we run out of glycogen, we must switch to fat instead, and as we said before, fat burns slower than carbs, so we will have to slow our pace.

- When we burn glucose, we inevitably make lactic acid, which causes fatigue. But, if we have more mitochondria, we can burn more fat at higher intensities. Burning fat does not produce lactic acid, so, fitter people have an improved ability to metabolize fat, sparing stored glucose, and delaying fatigue.

So, it is clear that the ability to deliver O_2 to the muscles is a key characteristic of being physically fit. In fact, we use this ability in one of the most accurate measures of aerobic fitness, called VO_{2max}. This is defined as the amount of O_2 that we can take from the air that we breathe and deliver to the muscles.

So, let's take a big-picture look at all the machinery we use in our body's supply chain:

- We need to have a respiratory system that can move a lot of air in and out quickly so that we can extract O_2 and get rid of CO_2.
- We need a lot of red blood cells (RBC) to carry O_2 to the muscles.
- To move the RBC, we need a strong pump (the heart) to circulate blood around the body, constantly delivering O_2, glucose, and fat to the muscles and removing CO_2 to be dropped off at the lungs.
- Finally, we need the muscles to be able to extract as much O_2 from the blood as possible so that we can run our aerobic pathways fast enough to prevent a shift to glycolysis, which will inevitably produce lactic acid.

Now let's look at the equation for VO_{2max} and see how each part changes with aerobic endurance training, one of the key health benefits of swimming for exercise:

$$VO_{2max} = HR_{max} \times SV_{max} \times A\text{-}V\,O_{2\,diff\,max}$$

Now, this looks much more complicated than it really is! Remember, VO_{2max} is a measure of O_2 delivery to the muscles. **HR_{max}** is pretty straightforward. It is our maximum heart rate measured in beats per minute (bpm). A typical resting HR for an untrained male is around 70 ml/beat. The faster the heart beats, the more blood it can circulate around the body. Endurance training reduces heart rate at rest and during all intensities of exercise that are below maximal. Think about how hard your heart was beating the first time that you swam a lap in your local pool. But, after a few weeks of swimming, covering that same distance in the same amount of time is not as hard, and your heart rate is lower. I'll explain how this happens when we get to SV_{max}. Interestingly, HR_{max} does not change with training. Your maximal heart rate has a ceiling that only changes with age. Starting around 30 years of age, the older you get, the lower your HR_{max}. This the biggest limiting factor to exercise performance in older people. As someone in his late 40's, I find this fact to be very distressing.

SV_{max} stands for maximal stroke volume, which is the volume of blood that gets pushed out of our heart, into circulation with each beat. Stroke volume is measured in milliliters of blood per beat. A typical resting SV for an untrained male is around 70 ml/beat. Endurance training rapidly increases stroke volume.

There are three factors at play here, and they occur at different times in the training process:

1. First, endurance training leads to an increase (10–20%) in the total volume of blood we have in our body. The impact of more blood volume is that the heart fills with more blood before each beat. Heart tissue has elastic properties, just like a water balloon. If you fill a water balloon, the rubber stretches. When you let go of the end of the balloon, it returns to its original size and squeezes out all the water. If you completely fill the balloon, you stretch it even more and it responds by squeezing out more water and squirting it a greater distance. The heart acts similarly. Although the balloon

is not actively pushing water like the heart does, stretching the heart tissue makes the cardiac cells contract much harder than they do when they're not stretched.

2. Next, in addition to having more blood volume, we make more RBC. This increases the total number of O_2 carriers. But here's the really interesting part, if we look at the hematocrit, that is the percentage of blood that is made of RBC vs. the liquid part of the blood (plasma), it actually goes down with training. This means that although we have more RBC, the amount of plasma increased even more. The result of this is thinner, less viscous blood. It is the perfect situation. We have increased the O_2 carrying capacity of the blood with more RBC, *and* made the blood thinner, and thus easier to move around the body and through the smallest blood vessels (capillaries) in our muscles, where gas exchange occurs. These changes to our blood volume and viscosity occur within weeks of beginning a new swimming program.

3. Finally, after several months of training, we start to see structural changes to the heart, it actually gets bigger.

When we multiply HR and SV, we get a metric called our cardiac output, which is represented by the letter Q, and is measured in liters of blood pumped around the body each minute.

The bigger the heart, the more blood it can pump out with each beat. This explains why both resting and submaximal HR decrease after training. Let's say that you are watching your favorite movie on the couch. Before beginning your new swimming program, your resting HR is 70 bpm. After six months of swimming regularly, you are back on the couch talking to a friend, but now your resting HR is only 60 bpm. Since rest is rest, your O_2 requirement is the same after training as it was before you began training (4900 ml/min). How did your resting HR decrease by 10 bpm? Since your SV increased, you get more blood out of your heart with each beat, so you require fewer beats to get the same amount of blood (and O_2) around the body.

Now that you understand what Q is, and the role it plays in fitness, let's look at the last factor for the VO_{2max} equation.

A-V O$_{2\text{ diff max}}$ is the volume of O_2 that our muscles take out of the blood as it passes through. There are three major players in *A-V O$_{2\text{ diff}}$*. The following list does not follow any rank or chronological order.

• Aerobic training leads to a significant increase in the number of capillaries (the smallest blood vessels) present in the muscles. This means that we have a much greater surface area available to deliver O_2, glucose, and fat, and remove CO_2 and lactic acid.

• Once the blood has perfused the muscles, we need to have a way of getting the O_2 off of the RBC and into the muscles. The solution is an iron rich, O_2 magnet called myoglobin. Aerobic training increases the amount of myoglobin present in the muscles, allowing them to extract more O_2 from the blood.

• Finally, now that we have gotten O_2 into the muscles, we had better have more furnaces to use it. That's exactly what happens. The number and size of the mitochondria increase dramatically with aerobic training.

These alterations in A-V O$_{2\text{ diff}}$ take months to years to complete, and it is important to point out that increasing A-V O$_{2\text{ diff}}$ does not change VO_{2max}. That is because the limiting factor to VO_{2max} is the size of the heart. We know this because when athletes have increased the number of RBC is circulation, either by transfusing additional blood into themselves, or by taking a hormone called EPO, to increase the number of RBC, VO_{2max} increases by as much as 10–12%. This means that the muscles already have plenty of extra space to take in and use extra O_2. It is our heart and circulatory system that limits O_2 delivery.

MITOCHONDRIA: OUR BODY'S POWERPLANTS

So, if increasing our A-V $O_{2\ diff}$ has no impact on VO_{2max}, why does it matter if it changes with training? The answer to that question lies with the little furnaces, the mitochondria. Remember that fat can only be metabolized in mitochondria. As we continue to train, our swimming pace gets faster. We don't "feel the burn" of lactic acid until swimming at much faster speeds than we could before. This is because we have shifted from burning mostly glucose at high intensities to burning a mixture of fat and glucose.

- The more fat we burn, the fewer carbs we burn.

- Less carb metabolism means we spare our glycogen stores. Remember, if we run out of muscle glycogen, we get fatigued.

- If we burn fat, we will not make as much lactic acid, which also delays fatigue.

Thus, although long-term endurance training does not improve our fitness in terms of O_2 delivery (VO_{2max}) beyond what happens after the first few months of training, it does dramatically improve our endurance at higher intensities of exercise. Not only that, but now that we have more fat-burning furnaces, we burn more fat all the time, at rest and during exercise. This changes body composition, and, assuming that you maintain a reasonable diet, leads to reduced fat-mass, and proportionally more lean mass.

Now, these are the three factors that we use to calculate VO_{2max}, and thus aerobic fitness. However, there are two additional peripheral systems that play major roles and are both impacted by aerobic endurance training:

- **The respiratory system** is responsible for moving air into and out of the lungs (ventilation) and interfacing with the circulatory system to allow for O_2 to enter the blood and CO_2 to leave. Of equal importance is the role that the respiratory system plays in maintaining the acid-base balance of the blood. Through a simple chemical reaction in the lungs, the removal of excess CO_2 from the blood during high-intensity exercise reduces acid levels in the blood and allows us to continue exercising. Aerobic training, and swimming specifically, improves the efficiency of our respiratory system.

- **Blood pressure** is the force that our blood exerts on the interior walls of the blood vessels. Think of it this way, if you fill up your garden hose with water, there will be a push outwards from the water trying to get out of the hose. We must maintain blood pressure in very strict boundaries. Too little is like having low water pressure in your house. You turn on the shower and get just a trickle of water. If blood pressure is too low, we cannot drive blood from our heart, deep into our muscles. Conversely, if the water pressure in your house is too high, you risk damaging your pipes. The same is true for our arteries. Too much blood pressure over time, leads to hardening of the arteries, which actually leads to even higher blood pressure. One of the many health benefits of aerobic exercise is reduced resting blood pressure. Swimming lowers blood pressure even more than either cycling or running, in most populations. Interestingly, merely standing in chest-deep water reduces blood pressure in the short-term. I will explain how this happens when we discuss the physical properties of water, and the physiological adaptations that occur when going to from land to an aquatic environment.

In summary, **physical fitness is the measure of how much O_2 we can deliver to our muscles during exercise**. Long-term, aerobic endurance training improves both our capacity to deliver O_2 and our capacity to use it to burn both glucose (and more importantly, fat) to make ATP. Assuming we eat a healthy diet, long-term training inevitably leads to changes in body composition, i.e., less body fat. But not all exercise is created equal. Swimming provides additional health benefits beyond what can be achieved with land-based exercises like running and cycling.

HUMAN PHYSIOLOGY AND AQUATIC ENVIRONMENTS

Being immersed in an aquatic environment, either partially or completely, feels much different than being on land. As you step into a pool, the water cradles and supports your body, almost lifting you off the ground. Your muscles lengthen and relax, your joints glide more smoothly through their ranges of motion, your heart rate slows, and it becomes easier to let your mind drift off to another place and time.

Buoyancy and Unloading the Body

Buoyancy is defined as an upward force exerted by water on an immersed object. Think about what happens when you slide into your bathtub. The water line rises higher and higher as more of your body is submerged. The volume of water that is displaced is equal to the volume of your body that is resting under the surface of the water. The more water that is displaced, the greater the upward force that is applied to body. Since the human body, on average is slightly less dense than is water, the force of buoyancy allows us to float, reducing the need for our muscles to maintain posture.

When standing in water up to the groin, approximately 40% of our body weight is unloaded from the knees and ankles. In navel-deep water, over 50% of body weight is unloaded. By the time you are in water up to the bottom of the sternum, with your arms at your side, 60% of your body weight is fully supported by the water, allowing your hips and lower back to relax. If you are brave enough to venture into neck deep water, only the weight of the head, 12–18 pounds, is acting as a compressive force that must be carried by the spine and neck muscles.

This makes water an ideal environment for exercise and rehabilitation when dealing with either chronic or acute musculoskeletal injuries or diseases. For example, athletic trainers and physical therapists often add water-based exercises like water-jogging or water-aerobics to the treatment regimen for fractures and sprains of the lower extremities, increasing blood flow to the area, and hastening the healing process. The buoyant properties of water allow for the injured joint or muscles to be isolated, eliminating the load of body weight. Treatment of back and spinal injuries often involves a combination of wearing flotation devices like water wings, floatation belts, or vests, and light weights on the ankles, effectively pulling the legs down and the torso up, elongating the spine and pelvic girdle. Under these conditions, blood flow to the tissues is significantly improved. This approach is often used with patients suffering from acute back injuries and degenerative forms of arthritis.

When you think of water-jogging and water-aerobics, you may envision a group of retirees, mostly women, gently floating around in a warm pool. But I can tell you from personal experience that water-jogging classes are no joke: even in waist-deep water, moving your body across the length of a 25-yard pool is a challenging endeavor. Water is around 55 *times* more viscous than is air, meaning that covering the same 25-yard distance on land costs a fraction of the energy as it does in water. Add in resistance devices—for example, water paddles that you hold in your hands while moving your arms back and forth—and you have a very tough workout.

Water-based exercises are often preferred for special populations who can't effectively support their own body weight during land-based exercise. Examples include the elderly suffering from sarcopenia, (muscle wasting associated with aging and a sedentary lifestyle), those with degenerative neuromuscular diseases such as multiple sclerosis, and Parkinson' disease, and developmental deficiencies, including cerebral palsy and autism spectrum disorder. Finally, overweight, and obese people often have severe limitations to the duration and intensity of exercise that they can do on land. Their muscles are already doing so much work to keep them erect that they simply can't work out as hard or as long a leaner person. In all these examples, the buoyant effects of water reduce the work of maintaining posture, allowing for more energy to be spent doing exercise.

CHAPTER 2

Swimming and Cardiovascular Health

The transition from a sedentary to active lifestyle brings several health benefits, none more important than the improved function of the cardiovascular system including the heart and all of the vessels through which blood flows. In popular health and fitness circles, the heart is often referred to as an engine, but this isn't an accurate analogy. In a car, the engine is where fuel is burned in the presence of O_2, converting chemical energy into mechanical energy, allowing the wheels to turn. As is always the case when converting energy from one form to another, the processes are not 100% efficient, generating heat that must be removed from the machine, be it a car engine, or a human body. From this description, it is obvious that the human equivalent of the engine are the muscles. This is where we burn our fuels, glucose and fat, in the presence of O_2, converting dietary nutrients into ATP, which provides the energy to move our muscles. Just like a car engine, we generate a lot of heat that must be removed, by radiation and sweating, or we will overheat just like a car.

So, what is the analogue for the heart? The heart does two jobs when it comes to exercise. It is the fuel pump that moves nutrients and O_2 to the muscles and removes excess heat and CO_2. To keep us cool during exercise, hot blood is moved from the interior of the body to the skin where the evaporative effects of sweating cool the blood. In this way, the cardiovascular system, along with the skin, work like a car radiator. To remove CO_2, the cardiovascular system pairs with the respiratory system to breathe it off, just like the tail pipe on a car. Although, all forms of aerobic endurance training improve cardiovascular health, swimming results in different adaptions to the heart, blood vessels, and even to the composition of the lipids (fat and cholesterol) that are transported in the blood, when compared to the most common forms of land-based training, i.e., running/walking and cycling.

SWIMMING AND VO$_{2MAX}$

The best and most used measure of aerobic fitness is VO_{2max}, the maximal volume of O_2 that your cardiovascular system can deliver to your muscles per minute during exercise (see Chapter 1 for more information). Let's assume that you are an average untrained, sedentary person who wants to start a new aerobic fitness routine tomorrow. If you trained appropriately, your VO_{2max} would increase rapidly, peaking after about 8–12 weeks. The way we test VO_{2max} is by putting you through a graded exercise test. This means you exercise at harder and harder intensities until you decide that you need to stop, we call this volitional exhaustion. Your exhaled air is captured in a mask, attached to a hose that leads to a gas analyzer, a device that measures the amounts of O_2 and CO_2 in the exhaled air. Since the amount of O_2 and CO_2 in the air that you inhale is constant, we can compare the composition of the inhaled air to the exhaled air to determine how much O_2 your body is extracting, and how much CO_2 you are producing.

Regardless of the type of exercise you do, the graded exercise test protocol is similar. The test is divided into a series of stages that are between

90 seconds and three minutes long. Subsequent stages get harder and harder, making you breathe deeper and faster, until you reach volitional exhaustion. Running tests use a treadmill, and as you progress from stage to stage, the speed and grade of the treadmill increase. During a cycling test resistance is added to the pedals, making you stamp down harder in order to keep moving at the same cadence. The old-school way to add resistance to a stationary bike was to hang weights from a strap attached to the front wheel, slowing its rotation. The modern method is to use what's called an electronically braked bicycle ergometer. A computer-controlled electromagnet clamps down on the wheel, making it harder to pedal.

Conducting a true graded exercise test in swimming is a bit more difficult. There are some field tests that allow you to swim in place while wearing a belt attached by pulleys, to a stack of weights. As more weight is added to the stack, it pulls you back to the wall. But wearing a weight belt can alter swim mechanics, reducing VO_{2max}, so, the best method requires the equivalent of a treadmill for swimming, called a flume. In a flume, water circulates through a small pool, into one end and out the other. The speed of the water flowing through the flume can be adjusted just like you would the speed of the belt on a treadmill. The speeds at which you swim during the test are converted to paces in yards/second or meters/second. As you can imagine, a flume is much more expensive than either a treadmill or a bicycle ergometer. Because of this, finding good research on the impacts of swimming on VO_{2max} is much tougher than finding studies on running or cycling. That said, these studies do exist.

Now, if you take one person and measure their VO_{2max} on a treadmill, and a bicycle ergometer, and then in a flume, you will likely get three different numbers. From highest to lowest, most people who are either untrained or moderately trained will record their highest VO_{2max} during running. Cycling VO_{2max} is typically second, with swimming third. This is because the total muscle mass used for each type of exercise is very different. The arms produce anywhere from 70–90% of the propulsive force of swimming during front crawl (Freestyle). Since cycling uses the legs, those large muscles require more O_2-rich blood to be delivered during exercise than do the arms. But the arm and core muscles do comparatively little work during cycling relative to running, so VO_{2max} is lower than in running. Running is a full weight bearing activity that requires all the major muscle groups to be actively engaged. The additional muscle mass recruitment increases the VO_{2max} achieved during a maximal graded exercise test. This is why running fitness does not translate to swimming fitness and vice versa.

For as long as I've been involved with athletics, I have heard people say that because swimming elicits a lower VO_{2max}, swimmers are less aerobically fit than are runners and cyclists. As is the case with most physiological systems, the truth is more nuanced than that. The genesis for this misconception is rooted in science. Studies from the 1970s tested elite athletes in different aerobic sports including swimming, cycling, running, cross-country skiing, and rowing for VO_{2max} using a graded running test on a treadmill. The runners and cross-country skiers frequently scored higher than the athletes from the other disciplines, but this was mostly a product of the study design.

If you test anyone for VO_{2max} in a discipline other their own, they will not perform as well as they would in their native sport. Years of practicing rowing with appropriate mechanics makes for a very efficient rower who will not fatigue as quickly as someone who has never pulled on oars before. I can tell you from personal experience that the first time I put my 6'3", 270-pound frame into a single shell, I spent most of my energy desperately trying not to fall into Lady Bird Johnson Lake. I didn't do very much rowing that day. Running, although it sounds like it should come rather naturally to all, is a very complex set of multi-joint movements that rowers, swimmers, and cyclists don't practice. But make no mistake—if you were to take a world class runner and drop them into a flume, I assure you that their VO_{2max} would be lower than that of a world class swimmer. More importantly, the runner's VO_{2max} during swimming would also be much lower than what they could accomplish on a treadmill. That said, at these levels of extreme fitness, there does appear to be a small, but statistically significant separation in VO_{2max} between cross-country skiers and all other athletes. This is likely the result of the combined effects of the amount of muscle mass used during skiing, and long-term training at high altitudes, which is known to increase the number of RBC in circulation.

As we drop down to the level of well-trained recreational athletes, the differences in aerobic fitness between sports disappears. Research on well-trained swimmers and triathletes, a race that involves swimming, cycling, and running in that order, shows that any measurable differences in VO_{2max} are the result of being more efficient in the native discipline. As a former triathlete, and current triathlon coach, I can attest to the fact that most triathletes spend the least amount of their training time in the pool. I often must nag my triathletes to complete their swimming sessions.

Evidence for this comes from a study during which VO_{2max} was measured in two groups of athletes, swimmers and triathletes[1]. Each athlete completed two graded exercise tests: one while swimming and the other while cycling. During the swimming tests, the swimmers outperformed the triathletes (58.4 vs. 51.3 ml/kg per minute). As expected, the triathletes outperformed the swimmers during the cycling test (68.2 vs. 53.0 ml/kg per minute). Again, it all comes back to mechanical efficiency in the exercise discipline. The triathletes likely spent more time training on the bike than in the pool and had better cycling mechanics than they did swimming mechanics.

More evidence for this comes in the fact that the maximal power output during the cycling test was significantly higher for the triathletes (350 vs 266.7 watts). Conversely, the swimmers' maximal swimming pace was significantly faster than that of the triathletes (1.36 vs. 1.21 m/s). Although the difference between the sport specific VO_{2max} and the swimmers and triathletes *looks* quite large, there was also a significant difference in age between the subjects; the swimmers were 16.1 years old on average, while the triathletes were 22.6 years old. An extra 6.5 years of physical development during the latter stages of adolescence makes an enormous difference when we consider the fact that the limiting factor of VO_{2max} is the size of the heart and the amount of blood in the body. In fact, the triathletes were 4.6 kg (10.2 lbs.) heavier than the swimmers.

So, we have established that the aerobic fitness of swimmers and other athletes is not different at the elite, and well-trained levels. But what about an untrained person who has just started swimming? A study from 1972 tested the VO_{2max} of elite swimmers, well-trained swimmers, and novice swimmers during swimming, cycling, and running[2]. Although the novice swimmers were "untrained" in regards of their swimming experience, they regularly participated in running and cycling. VO_{2max} measures for the elite and well-trained swimmers were the same during swimming, running, and cycling. But the novice swimmers had much lower VO_{2max} measures during swimming than during either cycling or running, and they made a lot more lactic acid. This means that swimming was much more stressful than either of the other two disciplines, resulting in the novice swimmers becoming fatigued more quickly. If the novice swimmers had a few months to train in a pool, using proper breathing technique, their swimming VO_{2max} would improve to match that of their cycling or running results.

So, the take-home message from all of this is that swimming stimulates similar adaptations in the cardiovascular system, e.g., increased heart size, increased blood volume, and greater mitochondrial capacity, as do either cycling or running. Now, let's shift our focus to how swimming impacts cardiovascular health.

SWIMMING AND CHRONIC HYPERTENSION

When you visit your doctor, they should always take your basic vital signs including resting blood pressure. If you've ever paid attention to your results, the doctor will report two numbers. Healthy blood pressure is usually around 120/80 mmHg. The top number is your systolic pressure, and the bottom number is your diastolic pressure. Systole is the phase of the cardiac cycle when the heart is squeezing blood out into circulation. If systolic pressure is too high, it may damage the walls of the arteries, reducing their elastic properties, making them stiffer and less compliant. Stiffer arteries lead to even higher blood pressure. If systolic pressure is too low, blood does not travel to all the tissues, a situation akin to having low water pressure in your house. You may notice this when blood pools in your legs after standing up too quickly. In this case, the blood pressure to your brain drops rapidly and you get dizzy for a moment.

Diastole is the phase of the cardiac cycle when the heart is relaxing and refilling with blood. This represents the residual pressure of the blood pushing on the arterial walls, without any influence from the heart. Diastolic pressure represents the backpressure of the blood pushing on the heart as it refills. If diastolic pressure is too high, the heart must generate more force to get blood out. An example would be like having a friend hold the front door closed as you are trying to exit a building. The more she pushes against the door, the harder you to have to push to open the door and get outside. If diastolic pressure is chronically elevated, the heart gets progressively weaker over time, until it stops pumping.

Because the maintenance of blood pressure is critical to survival, it is constantly monitored and adjusted by a complex mechanism of intertwined processes involving both the SNS, which rapidly controls HR and SV, and several hormones, that slowly control blood volume. Since this is a book about swimming, and not a medical text, we will only review the two most important elements of the blood pressure control system so that you can better understand how swimming alters our blood pressure regulation. We will start by discussing how the body responds to acute changes in blood pressure.

The central mechanisms of blood pressure control are receptors that detect changes in pressure, appropriately named baroreceptors (baro meaning "pressure"). We have two sets of baroreceptors:

- In the aorta, the main artery into which the heart pumps blood on its way to the body
- The carotid arteries leading to the brain

These locations were specifically chosen for good reason. Blood pressure is highest in the aorta because it is the systemic artery closest to the heart. The carotid arteries carry blood to the brain, the only organ that we cannot allow to go without blood for very long without dying. The baroreceptors send a constant stream of data about our blood pressure to the part of the brain stem that controls cardiovascular function. If adjustments to blood pressure are required, the instructions come from the brain stem.

Now that we have established the basic framework, let's set up two scenarios that will rapidly alter blood pressure, and see how the body responds in order to bring things back into balance. We will start with you lying on your couch watching TV for a few hours. In this horizontal position, blood is at the same level as the heart, increasing venous return, making it easier to fill the heart. If you stand up too quickly, the blood in your chest and abdomen pools in your legs and venous return decreases. Remember, less blood into the heart means less blood out of the heart, and arterial pressure drops quickly. You may feel light-headed and see stars. Your baroreceptors detect this drop in blood pressure and send a warning to the brainstem. The response is sent via the SNS to the heart and arteries. The heart responds by beating faster and harder, increasing cardiac output. The arteries vasoconstrict, squeezing on the blood, increasing pressure. After blood pressure stabilizes, you stop feeling woozy and can walk to the kitchen for a snack.

The second scenario starts with you standing straight and tall. You bend over to pick up something heavy from the ground, but before you lift it, you take a deep breath and hold it. This is called a Valsalva maneuver, and we all do this anytime we bear down or lift a heavy object. Holding your breathing fills your lungs with air, providing additional internal support for your back and abdominal muscles as they contract during the lift. The byproduct of this is a transient spike in blood pressure. The SNS responds by passively decreasing HR and SV, reducing cardiac output, and by vasodilating the arteries, reducing blood pressure.

Now that we have a basic understanding of how blood pressure is measured and adjusted in the short term, let's talk about the most common causes of chronic high blood pressure, hypertension. Chronic hypertension is associated with behaviors that increase blood volume and stiffness of the arteries. Excessive sodium intake makes us retain water in our circulatory system, which raises blood pressure. Diets high in fat and cholesterol, especially when combined with a sedentary lifestyle can lead to arterial plaque formation and stiffer, less compliant arteries, raising blood pressure.

Long-term aerobic endurance training reduces resting blood pressure by decreasing the SNS activity on the heart, and more importantly, on the blood vessels. In other words, training quiets the SNS and allows the Parasympathetic Nervous System (PNS) to have more input, resulting in a heart rhythm that is slower and less vigorous. The decreased SNS activity also leads to more vasodilation and less vasoconstriction of the arteries.

In general, all forms of aerobic exercise improve blood pressure to similar degrees, and there are no good studies that have made direct comparisons between swimming and land-based exercises in terms their respective abilities to regulate blood pressure. However, one study did compare the effects of participation in either water-based gymnastics or similar land-based exercises in patients undergoing rehabilitation for heart disease[3]. After three weeks of exercise and rehabilitation, the water gymnastics group experienced a non-significant decrease in both systolic pressure (119–109 mmHg), and diastolic pressure (71.7–65.7 mmHg). The authors provided two potential explanations for these changes.

The first was that the hydrostatic pressure of the water shifted blood from the lower extremities into the chest, increasing venous return and reducing the workload on the heart. This upward shift of blood volume also stretched the arteries, stimulating them to vasodilate. Another interesting result that supported the proposed mechanism was the fact that the water-gymnastics group experienced a significant increase in the circulating levels of a metabolite of nitric oxide (NO), a potent vasodilator that is produced by the cells that line the inside of the arteries.

As blood flow increases, the lining cells are stretched, stimulating them to release NO, causing the arteries to relax and vasodilate, increasing blood flow during exercise. Here is the kicker; the land-based exercise group experienced no changes in NO, systolic, or diastolic pressure.

The second potential explanation for the results was that exercising in chest-deep water unweighted the subjects, allowing them to use more of their cardiac output for exercise instead of maintaining posture. By contrast, the land-based group could not sustain the same workload for as long, reducing the total amount of exercise that could be done, significantly reducing the health benefits of the exercise session.

The headward shift of blood volume during water immersion temporarily increases blood pressure in the aorta and carotid arteries. I know this sounds counterintuitive but stay with me for just a few more sentences. With more blood in the chest and head, the baroreceptors tell the brain stem that there is extra fluid in the circulatory system that can be removed. The result is increased urine production, removing blood volume, and thus reducing pressure. When this process is repeated, the body reduces its total blood volume enough to lower resting blood pressure.

So, tying all of this together, the reduction of resting blood pressure after swimming is a multifactorial process:

- Swimming reduces basal SNS activity (less Fight or Flight), leading to lower heart rate and stroke volume, in other words, the heart beats slower and with less force.

- At the same time, PNS activity (Feed or Breed) increases, further lowering the cardiac output of the heart. These two effects are also observed after land-based training, but swimming may improve them even more.

- Water immersion shifts blood headwards, stretching the arteries, stimulating them to release NO, which causes arterial relaxation, and vasodilation.

- Lastly, the headward shift of blood transiently increases pressure in the arteries housing our baroreceptors, causing us to pee more, reducing blood volume, and thus, pressure. These last two effects are unique to swimming.

SWIMMING AND CHRONIC HYPOTENSION

Although the vast majority of those who suffer from chronic alterations in resting blood pressure are hypertensive, many people, particularly frail, elderly individuals suffer from chronically low blood pressure, or hypotension. If you will remember, most of our blood is in the venous side of our circulatory system at any given time because veins are larger and stretchier than are arteries. Additionally, unlike arterial blood, which is under relatively high pressure, venous blood pressure is as low as 0 mmHg in most instances. In order to get this blood back to the heart, we must rely on our leg muscles to squeeze on the veins as we walk, run, or ride a bike, pushing the blood back up to the heart. To prevent the blood from falling back down to our feet between contractions, there are a series of one-way valves in our veins that keep blood flowing in one direction, up. This system works very well in healthy people who are well hydrated, but as people age, particularly those who have been sedentary for many years, venous valves weaken and can fail to close. When weak, prolapsed venous valves are coupled with edema, dehydration, and a poor diet, low in protein, you have the perfect recipe for what's called orthostatic hypotension. This translates to low blood pressure when standing in the vertical position.

The treatments for orthostatic hypotension include exercise, and increased salt and water consumption to increase fluid retention. However, land-based exercise can be difficult because of low venous return to heart, reducing cardiac output. Because cardiac output is so severely reduced, these people have to exercise at reduced intensities for shorter durations, limiting the health benefits of exercise. This is where swimming is different. The hydrostatic pressure of the water, combined with switching positions from vertical to horizontal, provide two major benefits. First, the additional external pressure squeezes the veins, pushing blood toward the heart. Second, being in a horizontal position brings the blood level with the heart, reducing the influence of gravity. Both factors dramatically improve venous return to the heart, which increases cardiac filling, stretching the heart muscle, increasing stroke volume, and thus, the cardiac output. Swimming improves oxygen delivery in these people, allowing them to exercise at higher intensities for longer durations than could be achieved during land-based activity. Because of this, overall cardiovascular health improves significantly.

SWIMMING AND ALL-CAUSE MORTALITY RISK

Comparing forms of exercise for specific health benefits is a difficult task. Health outcomes typically take months to years to manifest, and most clinical studies only last a matter of weeks. In addition, in order to find statistically significant differences between groups, you need large numbers of subjects. Again, most clinical studies comparing swimming to land-based aerobic exercise involve relatively small sample sizes. However, one study conducted over 32 years looked at all-cause mortality rates in

40,547 men between the ages of 20-90 years[4]. Even after controlling for age, body-mass index (a standardized estimate of body fat), smoking status, alcohol consumption, and family history of cardiovascular disease, far fewer swimmers had died compared to sedentary controls (+53%), walkers (+50%), or runners (+49%). Of those who died during the study, the vast majority suffered at least one heart attack or stroke and suffered from hypertension and diabetes. The explanation for the results offered by the authors was that the total volume (duration of each session) and intensity of exercise in the swimming group were higher than for the walkers and runners. The reasons for this were the same as we have covered previously, swimming is easier on the musculoskeletal system of older, injured, or overweight/obese people, and reduces heat stress when compared to either walking or running.

In conclusion, swimming provides both indirect benefits to cardiovascular health, i.e., unweighting the body and reducing heat stress, and direct benefits, i.e., reduced SNS activity and improved vascular function, that land-based endurance exercises do not. Although any form of aerobic endurance exercise will improve cardiovascular function, there is ample evidence that swimming is the best prescription for a healthy lifestyle.

CHAPTER 3

Swimming and Pulmonary Health

THE BASICS OF BREATHING

The respiratory system has two functions: ventilation and gas exchange. **Ventilation** is the movement of air into and out of the lungs. Gas exchange is the movement of O_2 from the lungs into the circulatory system, and the removal of CO_2. Although there is ample evidence that aerobic endurance training increases the number of capillaries in the lungs, providing more surface area for gas exchange, there is no published data to suggest a difference between different types of exercise. However, several studies have shown that swimming improves ventilation more than does land-based endurance training.

Ventilation involves the inverse relationship between pressure and volume. As the pressure in the lungs decreases, the volume of the lungs increases, allowing air to rush into them. As the pressure in the lungs increases, the volume of the lungs decreases as the ribs and diaphragm squeeze air out of them. The movement of air during ventilation requires an extensive system of pipes that conduct air into and out of the lungs. These include the trachea, and bronchiole tubes that branch into smaller and smaller tributaries before reaching the alveoli, where gas exchange occurs. It is estimated that there are at least 30,000 bronchioles in each lung.

Like the arteries, the bronchioles are surrounded by a layer of smooth muscle that controls the volume of air that flows through by bronchoconstriction and bronchodilation. Finally, in order to moisten the air as it moves into the lungs, and remove any allergens or pathogens, the bronchiole tubes produce a thin layer of mucus that traps particulate matter. Once captured in the mucus, the foreign material is swept back up to the mouth and sinuses by cilia that produce a constant current, flowing upward, away from the lungs. As a last stand against infection of the lungs, the bronchioles may become inflamed, severely restricting ventilation until the immune system can clear the foreign particles.

Ventilation is divided into **inspiration** (inhalation) and **expiration** (exhalation). We can further classify each process as either resting or forced (as occurs during exercise). Resting inspiration involves the external intercostals, which lift the ribs up and out, and the diaphragm, which contracts down into the abdominal cavity, making more space in the chest. Both actions increase the volume of the lungs, reducing air pressure, allowing air to flow in. Resting expiration is a passive process. The external intercostals and diaphragm relax, returning to their original positions, while the elastic properties of the lungs themselves, recoil to their original, unstretched shape. Both actions reduce the volume of the lungs, increasing the pressure in the lungs, forcing air out.

As exercise intensity increases, we experience an internal drive to increase ventilation, forced inspiration and expiration. During the transition from rest to moderate intensity exercise, increased ventilation is driven by the need for more O_2. But, as we move from moderate to high-intensity exercise, increased ventilation is driven by the need to remove CO_2 as rapidly as possible in an attempt to maintain the acid-base balance of the blood. In order to ventilate more air during exercise, additional muscles are recruited to increase the rate and depth of ventilation. The objective of forced inspiration is to pull the rib cage up even further, expanding lung volume, reducing lung pressure, drawing in more air. Think about what you do with your arms after you have finished a fast run and you are trying to catch your breath. You either put hands behind your head with your elbows bent, or your put your hands on your waist and jut your hips forward. Both positions increase lung volume, making it easier to inhale. The pectorals and two sets of neck muscles contract to assist in lifting the ribs up even further during peak ventilation. The objective of forced expiration is to squeeze even more air out of the lungs than happens during resting expiration. To do this, the internal intercostal and several muscles that bring the hips and shoulders closer together contract, reducing lung volume, increasing pressure, and forcing air out. These include the abdominals, the lats, and muscles that attach the lower ribs to the pelvis. In conjunction with the increased respiratory muscle activity during exercise, the SNS stimulates bronchodilation, allowing a greater volume of air to move in and out faster.

Aerobic exercise improves the endurance of these respiratory muscles, making them more efficient and fatigue resistant. But swimming adds the element of external resistance as the hydrostatic pressure of the water pushes against the ribs as they are contracting outward. Just like what happens to arm or leg muscles after resistance training, the respiratory muscles get stronger.

The other difference between land-based exercises and swimming is that unlike running and walking, during which you can breathe continuously, you must hold your breath when swimming. In doing so, O_2 delivery to the muscles is reduced when compared to land-based exercise. This creates a hypoxic environment in which less ATP can be made aerobically. The difference must be made up by glycolysis, which produces lactic acid. Acidic blood is a potent stimulator of the respiratory centers in the brain stem, resulting in significant increases in breathing depth and speed.

Pulmonary Function Test

A pulmonary function test measures both the volume and speed with which we move air in and out of the lungs. Like a VO_{2max} test, you wear a mouthpiece connected by a hose to a device called a spirometer that measures both the rate of flow and the volume of air moved. To keep air from escaping through your nose, you also wear a nose clip. The test is conducted in the seated position at rest. After taking 5 to 10 normal breaths, you are instructed to fill your lungs with as much air as you can, as quickly as possible. This is a forced, maximal inspiration. Immediately after you reach your peak volume, you are instructed to blast all the air out as fast as you can. This is a forced, maximal expiration. The test is finished when your normal breathing rhythm and depth are restored. This simple test measures several variables, each revealing something about your respiratory health.

Tidal Volume (TV). This is the volume of air that moves in and out with each normal breath at rest. On the readout of a pulmonary function test, TV looks like a series of waves with the crests being inspiration and the troughs being expiration.

Inspiratory Reserve Volume (IRV). This is the extra volume that is inhaled, above the crest of the TV, during a maximal inspiration. The total volume and the speed of the IRV tell us how strong the inspiratory muscles are, and whether there are any obstructions in the airways, like mucus, inflammation, or bronchoconstriction.

Expiratory Reserve Volume (ERV). This is the extra volume exhaled, below the trough of the TV, during a maximal expiration. The total volume and speed of the ERV tell us how strong the expiratory muscles are, whether or not there are any obstructions, and if the elastic property of the lung tissue is impaired.

Vital Capacity (VC). This represents the total volume of air that can be moved in and out of the lung. You can never get all the air out of your lungs. That would result in a collapsed lung. So, there is always some air left in the lungs at the end of a forced, maximal expiration. This is called the residual volume (RV). Residual Volume cannot be measured during a pulmonary function test. But it can be estimated. Measuring RV requires a different test. When we add all these volumes together, we get Total Lung Capacity (TLC). Elevated TLC is associated with better aerobic fitness.

Forced Expiratory Volume in 1 second ($FEV_{1.0}$). This is the volume of air that can be exhaled in the first second of a forced, maximal expiration.

Peak Expiratory Flow Rate (PEFR). This is the greatest rate of flow of air out of the lungs during a forced, maximal expiration.

Both the $FEV_{1.0}$ and the PEFR provide additional information about potential obstructions of air flow that the IRV and ERV do not. Perhaps a patient can move a normal volume of air, but it take a very long time. A lower peak flow or $FEV_{1.0}$ show us that air is moving very slowly, perhaps through restricted airways.

Maximal Inspiratory Pressure (MIP) and Maximal Expiratory Pressure (MEP). These are akin to a one-rep max for the respiratory muscles and tell us how much force they can generate in one contraction. Both of these flow and pressure measures improve dramatically after aerobic, endurance training.

SWIMMING AND PULMONARY FUNCTION

Studies dating back to the 1960s have conclusively shown that swimming is superior to land-based exercise when it comes to improving pulmonary function. In one such study, measures of VC, $FEV_{1.0}$, and PEFR of young men competing in soccer, field hockey, basketball, volleyball, and swimming were compared to each other and a sedentary control of similar age[1]. Although all the active groups had significantly higher values for all three measures than did the control group, the swimmers' measures were significantly higher than any of the land-based athletes. The authors explained these results as being the product of three factors:

1. Exercising in a horizontal position during swimming increases the stress on the respiratory muscle when compared to exercise in the vertical position. Try breathing while lying on your belly, face down. Now try again, but this time with your head cocked up so that you're looking straight ahead at the wall. It is much tougher to breathe with your head in this position. Even if you turn your head sideways as you would during freestyle swimming, this is still more difficult than breathing when your head is in a neutral position, i.e., in line with your spine.

2. The external force on the abdominal and thoracic cavities generated by the hydrostatic pressure of water.

3. The increased production of lactic acid as a result of hypoxia during swimming.

These adaptations have been observed in children as young as seven years old! Maximal inspiratory pressure and MEP were measured in 75 children between 7–8 years, who participated in either swimming or indoor soccer, or were in the sedentary control group[2]. Although there was no difference in either measure between the soccer players and the controls, the swimmers had significantly faster flow rates than either of the other groups.

Since none of these children suffered from any respiratory diseases, the improved flow rates were attributed to stronger respiratory muscles as a result of swimming. In this case, the authors added one more possible explanation for the results. Swimming requires the use of muscles that move the arms, trunk, and head, including the lats, abdominals, pectoral, and two neck muscles: the scalenes and sternocleidomastoids. All these muscles are also respiratory muscles; they effectively pull double duty during swimming that doesn't occur to the same degree during land-based exercise. Swimming improves the function of these muscles for both swimming *and* breathing at the same time.

A subsequent study conducted in India found that not only does swimming improve pulmonary function more than land-based exercise, but also these changes are cumulative over many years of swimming[3]. The authors compared VC, IRV, TV, and $FEV_{1.0}$ in four groups of men between the ages of 20-45 years. The four groups were:

1. A group of non-swimming controls who were not participating in any exercise.
2. A group who had been swimming for less than two years.
3. A group that had been swimming between 2–5 years.
4. A group that had been swimming for more than five years.

All swimming groups practiced two hours a day, five days a week. In the first two years of swimming, there were no changes when compared to the control group. However, after two years there were significant changes in each measure, and after five years of swimming, all four measures increased further still. Clearly the rate of change in these older subjects was not as rapid as was observed in the children, but the fact that these changes to pulmonary function happened at all in older populations is impressive. So, as they say, it's never too late to start swimming! Okay, no one says that but me, but it's going to catch on.

As amazing as the results of the previous study are, they pale in comparison to the next study. Researchers wanted to see if the adaptations to pulmonary function go away after we stop swimming[4]. They followed a group of 30 female swimmers (12–16 years old) over seven years from 1961–1968, measuring pulmonary function every 2.5 years. After seven years, none of the subjects were swimming any longer, but their pulmonary function had largely remained stable. When controlling for increases in height (over seven years, teenagers get taller), measures of VC, RV, and TLC all stayed the same or increased slightly. When we combine these results with those of the Indian study we see that swimming, over many years, molds the pulmonary system, expanding its functional capacities, and these adaptations can last for at least several years after swimming stops.

Now, I'm not suggesting that swimming for 5–10 years and then doing nothing is all you need to do to protect yourself from the ills of a sedentary lifestyle thereafter. But clearly, swimming leads to physiological adaptations that have lasting benefits even when you no longer put on your trunks.

SWIMMING AND ASTHMA

Asthma is a chronic respiratory disease that results in bouts of acute bronchoconstriction. An asthma attack is often described as feeling like you're breathing through a drinking straw. The underlying causes include genetics, and chronic exposure to environmental irritants such as smoking, dust, exhaust fumes, or other chemicals. Additional risk factors for developing asthma include having allergic conditions like dermatitis and hay fever and being overweight or obese. There are three types of asthma:

1. Occupational asthma that is triggered by irritants specific to your workplace, e.g., airborne chemicals or dusts.

2. Allergy-induced asthma triggered by particulate matter including pollen, mold, cockroach droppings, and pet dander.

3. Exercise-induced asthma, which is the least understood, but is frequently made worse by exercise in cold, dry environments.

Although there is some evidence that long-term exposure to chlorine in swimming pools can lead to mild forms of asthma in a small subset of swimmers[5], the overwhelming consensus is that swimming significantly improves respiratory function and reduces the need for medical therapeutic treatments for symptoms in both children and adults. Since obesity is a risk factor for developing asthma, exercise is an important supplemental treatment. But land-based exercises pose several barriers including weight-bearing, heat stress, and breathing cold, dry air. As we have covered, swimming unloads the body, dissipates heat quickly, and provides warm, moist air to breathe, all while strengthening respiratory muscles, which are already weakened by a lack of exercise as a result of having asthma.

Swimming has been shown to improve aerobic capacity in asthmatic children (8–12 years) during both swimming and cycling tests[6]. Two groups of asthmatic children (a swimming group and non-exercise control group) were tested before and after six weeks (seven days a week) of high-intensity swimming at 125% of the intensity that increased lactic acid levels in the blood (lactate threshold, LT). The training sessions consisted of two 15-minute bouts of continuous swimming with a 10-minute break in between. Before and after the six-week training period, both groups completed two graded exercise tests, one swimming, and another on a cycle ergometer. They defined aerobic capacity as the speed the subjects could swim (or ride) before lactic acid started to accumulate in the blood.

Remember that aerobic endurance training increases the intensity of exercise that can be sustained before lactic acid floods into the circulation by increasing the use of fat instead of glucose. During the swimming test, the swimming group experienced an increase in their aerobic capacity of approximately 24%, while the control group had a non significant increase of only 4%. Interestingly, swimming improved aerobic function during cycling as well (approx. 24%), while the control group experienced a non-significant increase (approx. 10%). The authors chose a swimming protocol at 125% of LT because this would fully stimulate the SNS (fight or flight) response, simulating bronchodilation. It appears that in order to reap the full benefits of swimming, asthmatics need to swim at high intensities that require the use of both the aerobic and anaerobic energy pathways.

Another study found similar results. Asthmatic children completed three months of swim training at their LT, followed by another three months of high-intensity training above their LT[7]. These children experienced dramatic improvements in VO_{2max} and HR_{max} that could be achieved during a graded cycling exercise test before fatigue. But what was more interesting was that while the total volume of air breathed in and out each minute (minute ventilation) increased after the swim training, the total number of breaths taken per minute did not. That means that each breath was deeper after swim training, exactly what you would want if you suffered from asthma. Breathing efficiency improved dramatically because of the combined effects of less bronchoconstriction and stronger respiratory muscles. None of these changes were observed in the control group of asthmatic children who did not train over the six months of the study.

When someone has an asthma attack, the total amount of air that they can take in with each breath decreases because their bronchiole tubes have constricted. In order to maintain the same minute ventilation, they must increase their respiratory rate, meaning they hyperventilate. This significantly reduces their capacity for exercise, not only because they can't move as much air, but also because their respiratory muscles fatigue more quickly.

Children who participated in three months of swim training at their LT experienced much less hyperventilation after training, and the degree of improvement was greater in those with the most obstructed breathing at the beginning of the study[8]. So, the benefits of swimming are scalable, those with worse asthma improve more than those with less severe asthma. But the best part is that regardless of where you start on the spectrum, you end up at levels close to non-asthmatics after swim training.

As we covered in the previous section, the benefits of swimming on pulmonary function in otherwise healthy people may last for years, even after participation in swimming has ended. There is evidence that the same is true for asthmatics. One study demonstrated that just two months of swimming (one hour, three days a week) improved pulmonary function and reduced the frequency and severity of asthma symptoms[9]. Measures were taken before and immediately after the two months of training, and a year after the subjects stopped swimming. The results of the swimming group were compared to those of a control group that did not participate in any exercise intervention.

A year after the swimming sessions concluded the swimming group experienced 78% fewer asthma attacks (control was only -11%), 89% fewer trips the emergency room (control was only -13%), and the number of days of school missed decreased by 82% (control was only -17%). Peak flow rates also remained significantly improved compared to before the swimming sessions, increasing by 65% at six months and staying at 63% after a year. The control group saw smaller changes that were attributed to growth, 21% at six months and 25% after a year, respectively. Clearly, swimming not only improves pulmonary function and exercise performance in asthmatics, but their quality of life as well. Best of all, these improvements are long lasting, extending for at least a year after participation in swimming had ceased.

CHRONIC OBSTRUCTIVE PULMONARY DISORDER (COPD)

Unlike asthma, which is primarily caused by obstructed breathing into the lungs, COPD primarily reduces airflow *out* of the lungs, leaving the subject feeling as though they can't empty their lungs. The two most common conditions that contribute to COPD are chronic bronchitis and emphysema. During chronic bronchitis the bronchiole tubes become chronically inflamed. Emphysema is scarring of the lung tissue, reducing its elastic properties, preventing air from the leaving the lungs. Treatment of COPD includes aerobic exercise training in combination with pulmonary rehabilitation. Although land-based exercises are most commonly prescribed because of accessibility, most people with COPD are elderly and suffer from numerous comorbidities including musculoskeletal injury or disease, cerebrovascular disease, and obesity. These frailties limit their ability to participate in land-based exercise training at high intensities, and result in high rates of attrition, reducing their effectiveness in the treatment of COPD. So, what's the solution? Swimming, of course!

As we have seen several times now, the aquatic medium reduces the external stresses of weight bearing and heat accumulation. But there is a bonus to exercising in water when you suffer from COPD, the hydrostatic pressure helps you exhale. Remember that COPD is a disease of the lungs that restricts exhalation, so an aquatic hug helps squeeze more air out of the lungs.

In a 2013 study, 53 subjects who were participating in outpatient pulmonary rehabilitation for COPD were recruited, and randomly assigned them to one of three groups: water-based exercise, land-based exercise, or a non-exercise control group[10]. The exercise protocol was water aerobics. The intervention period lasted 12 weeks and consisted of three, 60-minute sessions per week. The pulmonary function measures were MIP and MEP. The subjects were also tested for their walking endurance with a self-paced six-minute walk test (6MWT) for distance, and two shuttle tests; the Endurance Shuttle Walk Test (ESWT) and Incremental Shuttle Walk Test (ISWT). During each test, the subjects walked down and back between two cones placed ten meters apart. The pace of the ESWT was fixed, while the ISWT got progressively faster. The subjects continued until they became fatigued. Finally, the subjective feelings of general fatigue, anxiety, and depression were assessed by questionnaire.

The retention rate of the subjects in the water-based training (83%) was higher than that of the land-based group (75%). The water-aerobics group outperformed the land-based exercise group in all three exercise tests, subjective measures of fatigue, labored breathing, emotional well-being, and MIP. Interestingly, when compared to land-based exercises, water-based exercises improved endurance during the ESWT (228 meters farther than control) and the ISWT (39 meters farther than control). The level of self-reported general fatigue was also lower in the water-aerobics group compared to the land-based exercise group.

On average, all subjects were elderly (>70 years) and obese (>30 BMI), making weight bearing activities and heat-dissipation more difficult for the land-based exercise group than for those in the water-aerobics group, limiting the intensity and duration of the exercise that could be completed during the intervention. Although there was no difference in MIP between the two exercise groups, the water-aerobics group did experience a significant improvement relative to the control group while the land-based group did not. This suggests that exercise in an aquatic environment, with the extra resistance of hydrostatic pressure, increases the strength of the inspiratory muscles to a greater degree than does land-based exercise.

CYSTIC FIBROSIS AND SWIMMING

Cystic fibrosis (CF) is a hereditary disease of the respiratory and digestive systems. The underlying cause is a recessive genetic mutation that results in the production of extremely thick mucus that clogs the bronchioles tubes, making ventilation difficult, and increasing the risk of respiratory infections. Exercise is a critical part of treatment as it allows the patients to break up the mucus and remove it. Unfortunately, many patients understandably reduce their regular physical activity, leading to muscle wasting, and further disease progression. As we have seen before, water-based activities, including swimming, provide additional physical support and less heat stress. Another benefit is the fact that exercise is taking place in a humid environment, particularly when in indoor pools. The inhaled water vapor loosens the mucus. By contrast, exercise in dry, cold air, significantly increases mucus production, making exercise more stressful.

Twelve weeks of swimming, three days a week for 60 minutes a session, in warm water (32°-35° C, 89.6°-95° F) significantly improved endurance during a treadmill walking test (+14%), VO_{2max} (+27%), and maximal minute ventilation (+15%), in a group of young children (~10 years of age) with CF[11]. An age-matched, non-exercise control group saw no changes over the same time period. The parents of the children in the swimming group reported that their children were able to cough up much more mucus in the hours after a swimming session then they normally did after a respiratory therapy session.

Although all forms of aerobic-endurance training improve pulmonary function in both healthy people and those suffering from chronic respiratory diseases, swimming offers unique benefits. Hydrostatic pressure provides support, reducing the effects of gravity on the body, allowing for that extra energy that usually goes to weight bearing, to be used to conduct exercise at higher intensities for longer durations. In other words, the quality of the workout is improved when you exercise in an aquatic environment. The external pressure makes our inspiratory muscles work harder to move air in, making them more efficient. Finally, the temperature of the water, either cool (reduced heat stress) or warm (increased mucus clearance) improves the exercise experience as well.

CHAPTER 4

Swimming and Bone Health

My favorite analogy for bone is concrete. Both have tough exteriors composed of minerals that provide compressive strength, with concrete being made of cement and bone being made of hydroxyapatite. You can stack blocks of cement very high without losing structural integrity. But, if a stiff wind blows, or the ground under the foundation moves, the structure will begin to twist and bend. These tensile and shear forces will eventually break the cement, and your tower of blocks will come tumbling down. To prevent this, engineers add in a latticework of interconnected steel rebar that can resist all the twisting, pulling, and bending. Similarly, hydroxyapatite is laid down over an inner structure of collagen fibers that provide resistance against the pulling and twisting that we do when we move.

Bone formation begins during fetal development *in utero*. Bones start as cartilage and are slowly converted into bone. After birth, bones continue to grow, and change in shape and size until our early 20s when our growth plates fuse. But even after we are no longer growing taller, modification to bone continues. Exercise leads to additional bone being made, thickening them. By contrast, when we stop exercising for long stretches, the extra bone material is removed because it is metabolically costly to keep material that we don't need. As they say, "Use it or lose it."

Changes in bone structure throughout life occur through one of two related processes called bone modeling and bone remodeling. To explain these processes, I will use an analogy of your bones being like your house. The original structure was made when it was first built; this is modeling. Now that you have lived in the house for several years, you've noticed that it has accumulated some wear and tear, and you may want to remodel the home. Bones are the same. We model our bones throughout our youth and adolescence. Once our growth plates are fused, all other changes are remodeling, either adding or removing bone. Both modeling and remodeling require two specialized cells, osteoblasts that lay down new bone, and osteoclasts, that remove bone.

During primary ossification *in utero*, osteoblasts lay down collagen and hydroxyapatite until they become trapped inside the new bone. At this point they change into "bone cells" called osteocytes. Osteoblasts that are on the outside (or inside the marrow cavity) of the bone when bone formation stops, go into a state of hibernation, and change into lining cells, because they line the surfaces of the bones. Although osteocytes no longer make bone, they maintain a very important function to bone health. The osteocytes are connected to all their neighboring osteocytes, and can relay signals throughout the entire bone, and potentially to other cells in the body. These signals are sent in response to the amount of "load" that is on the bone at any given time. Now, the term load is not entirely understood, but what is known is that gravity plays a major role in maintaining bone health, particularly in the weight-bearing bones of the legs, pelvis, and vertebrae.

Daily activities like standing, walking, and lifting everyday items like kids and groceries, adds enough load to the bones to keep them strong and healthy. But, if we add additional loads, beyond what the bones are used to handling, small, microfractures appear. If this were to happen in a wall of your home, and you just slapped some Spackle and paint over the top, it would cover the damage, but it wouldn't fix it. Over time that crack would grow, and the wall may fail and bring down the whole house with it. The same principle applies to bone. The microfractures stimulate the osteocytes to call in the repair crew. This starts with the accumulation of the demolition team, osteoclasts. These are huge cells that release digestive enzyme and acids onto the damaged bone to remove all the material in the microfracture zone. Once the debris is cleared there is a pit left behind. The lining cells surrounding the pit come out of their slumber and become osteoblasts again, making new bone, and repairing the damaged area. This process of damage-demolition-repair is called bone remodeling, or bone turnover, and we do it throughout life.

If the extra load that caused this remodeling only happens once, then there will be no need for extra bone to be made. But, if you start to do exercises that chronically add more than the usual load, e.g., running, or weightlifting, the osteocytes recognize that the bone does not have the appropriate density to sustain this new activity, in other words, the load is too much for the bone that you have. The solution is to add more, new bone, into the same volume that the old bone occupied. More material in the same volume means that bone mineral density increases. When bone remodeling results in denser bones, the osteoblasts are more active than the osteoclasts.

The process runs in reverse when we become sedentary. If you decide to stop running or lifting weights, your bones will experience less load. Since bone is metabolically costly tissue, if you don't use it, you will lose it. The long bones of your arms and legs won't shrink, but they will become less dense over time as the osteoclasts remove more bone than is laid down by the osteoblasts. Unfortunately, the same process happens as we age, and if we combine aging with a sedentary lifestyle, we get a double-whammy of bone wasting, or osteopenia. If this osteopenia continues unchecked, the vertebrae begin to deform under the weight of the upper body, height decreases, and the spine may arch, producing a hunched posture. These are the classic signs of osteoporosis, a disease state in which the bone mineral density is so low that there is an increased risk of fracture. Of greatest concern is the increased risk of fractures to the hips. The one-year mortality rate of those who fracture their hip is 22%[1]. Think of how many lives could be saved, and how many more who could have a better quality of life, if they only exercised as little as 20 minutes a day.

One of the most frequently cited studies about the effects of swimming on bone mineral density (BMD), relative to other sports[2], compared the BMD in the heel bone of three groups of adolescent female athletes including swimmers, soccer players, and weightlifters. All athletes had been participating in their respective sports for around five years and had similar training loads in terms of hours/weeks and months/year. The soccer players had the highest BMD in the heel bone, and the difference between them and the swimmers was statistically significant. To answer the question of whether or not the reduced BMD of the swimmers put them at greater risk of injury, the authors compared the data to normative values for regularly active, but not athletic, adult females (25 years old) collected by the World Health Organization (WHO)[3].

Both the soccer players and weightlifters had significantly higher BMD than the WHO normative values, while the swimmers were significantly lower. But this data must be taken with a really big grain of salt. The swimmers were also much younger (12 years old) than either the soccer players (15.1 years) or the weightlifters (13.6 years). Separate from the effects of any exercise activity, an extra 1.5-3 years of development during adolescence significantly increases BMD. Between the ages of 10–20 years[4], BMD increases at a rapid rate from approximately 0.82–1.09 g/cm^3. By contrast, average BMD peaks at around 1.13 g/cm^3 at around age 35. So, comparing the BMD of developing teenage girls to 25-year-old women (BMD ~ 1.1 g/cm^3) is apples to oranges. It is very likely that a follow-up study on these same swimmers would show that they grew into women with normal, healthy bones, at no greater risk for injury than anyone else. So, although weight-bearing activities like soccer and weightlifting increase BMD more than does swimming, swimmers still have very strong, healthy bones.

SWIMMING AND BMD

There is little question that exercise, in general, improves BMD. But not all exercise is created equal. When comparing long-duration, endurance exercise to sprint activities, we see a clear difference in BMD in both runners and swimmers[5]. When 52 males aged 17-30 years old (21 runners, 16 swimmers, and 15 controls) were examined for whole body and lower-leg BMD, the swimmers and runners who were categorized as sprinters had significantly higher BMD at all sites than did the endurance athletes. This is likely the combination of two factors:

- Sprinting generates much greater forces in the muscles that pull on the bones. These greater forces are load, that simulates bone turnover and growth.

- The second factor is related to nutrition. Endurance athletes spend much more time training and tend to eat less than their sprinting peers. More energy expenditure, combined with reduced food intake, impairs the body's capacity to recover between workouts. Limiting the volume of nutrients, namely protein, needed to repair broken down bones, is a major problem in aerobic, endurance athletes.

It has been found that drinking two smoothies of whey protein (you can buy this at any grocery store) at two and five hours after a high-intensity swimming workout significantly improved markers of bone formation and reduced signs of bone breakdown[6]. These changes didn't happen when the swimmers drank a carbohydrate rich smoothie, or water.

So, what have we learned?

- The weight-bearing nature of land-based exercises may provide a greater stimulus for bone growth than does swimming in some populations. But these differences are minimal, and the BMD of swimmers is certainly not low enough to increase the risks of skeletal injury.

- Including high-intensity sprinting may reduce this difference even more.

- Eating or drinking small amounts (15 grams) of protein shortly after a swimming workout has been shown to stimulate bone growth and prevent excessive breakdown.

All forms of exercise improve bone health. Swimming appears to at least keep pace with other forms of land-based exercise when it comes to stimulating increased bone mineral density, and when we consider that many long-time runners suffer from osteoarthritis and other over usage injuries associated with high impact forces, the balance is still heavily tipped in the favor of swimming as the best form of exercise to improve and maintain bone health.

CHAPTER 5

Swimming for Weight Loss and Weight Management

One of the reasons that my mother started me in swimming in the first place was because I was not gaining weight, having lost much of my appetite after my parents' divorce. Thankfully, one of her friends told her about how her kids would plow through their meals as if they hadn't eaten in days after every swim practice—and to my mother's great relief, I did the same. Unlike my eating habits after soccer or track practice, when I would pick at my food, after a session in the pool, I devoured my dinner and woke up with a healthy appetite the next morning. In short order, my weight had stabilized, and I was thriving again.

Later on, while working as an exercise physiologist in training, I started wondering why swimming was so different in terms of its impact on my appetite. I started to keep a food journal of the types and quantities of food that I ate on my swim days and compared them to my running and cycling days, and found I typically consumed 5–10% more calories during the meal immediately after my swimming sessions compared to the other two training days. Yet for the rest of the day, I tended to eat about the same, sometimes even a little less. When I asked my other triathlon friends if they experienced the same differences in appetite, most of them confirmed that they did. The few who did not, swam in mixed-use pools, e.g., swim lessons for little kids, or rehabilitation pools used by the elderly or injured, that had to be kept between 88–90°F, much warmer than the competition temperature of the pools that I was swimming in (around 77°F).

As an experiment, I joined one of my friends at his community indoor pool and found it to be a *miserable* workout. Although it felt great jumping in the warm water, before we had finished the warm-up, I could feel myself sweating, something I only experienced when swimming outdoors in the summer. After the session was done, I felt sleepy, almost woozy. I had no appetite for a few hours thereafter, and even then, I only picked at my meal without any real pleasure. To make matters worse, I was so hot! I had the AC set at 68°F and the ceiling fan on full tilt all night long. I tried this a few more times at my friend's warm pool, with the same results each time, although I did seem to adjust to it a bit more after each workout.

To extend this experiment a bit further, I asked around to see if anyone had access to a particularly cold pool. This resulted in a weekend trip down to Barton Springs, a spring-fed pool that maintains a year-round temperature of around 68°F. Jumping in is a shock and if you don't get moving quickly you may start to shiver.

To keep the variables of the experiment as close to what I did with the hot pool workouts, I slept in Austin the night before, ate the same meals for dinner and breakfast as I did before the hot swims, swam at the same time of day, and did the same workout. The difference was amazing. I was already feeling peckish at the end of the warm-up; before the 90-minute workout was done, *I was ready to eat!* I made it to the parking lot and dug into my lunch, eating everything that I brought and extra (as I had planned for this possibility). The result was that I had eaten 13% more calories than I would normally eat after a swim in my 77°F "normal" pool. Two hours later, I ate another small meal. For the entire day I was over my normal consumption by about 7%. Clearly ambient temperature and thermal control were the key issues here.

IMPORTANCE OF WATER TEMPERATURE

So, what is the reason for all this? The answer is that water conducts heat much more efficiently than does air. When we exercise in colder water, not only do we have to burn carbs and fat to move through the water, but we also have to make extra heat to keep us warm enough to function. The same is true when we run or cycle on land. There is a temperature sweet-spot (around 64–70°F) where we dissipate the heat of exercise in balance with the environment. At these temperatures we neither need to make extra heat to stay warm, nor do we absorb extra heat from the environment that we need to shed by sweating excessively. This is why all the major, non-Olympic marathons are run in the late-fall through early-spring months.

So, you must be asking at this point, "Why does this matter?" That's a good question. Around the same time as I was experimenting on myself, I started coaching triathlon. Many of my athletes, typically women who were new to the sport and had the least experience with swimming, started telling me anecdotal reports about how swimmers had higher amounts of body fat than did other athletes. They were concerned that swimming could make them gain extra fat. I knew that my body composition had changed when I went from only swimming to triathlon. I went from about 14% body fat at my leanest as a swimmer at 21 years old, to about 10% at my leanest as a 34-year-old triathlete. But I also had a much better diet in my 30's than I did in college. I didn't drink as much, or stay up late partying as often, etc.

Because, I didn't have a solid answer for my new athletes, I started digging a little deeper. The research was clear: swimming, particularly in colder water, will increase your food intake compared to running or cycling, but that does not lead to extra weight gain, because you also burn more calories in the form of extra heat that is generated by your body to stay warm. If there is a change in body composition that occurs after starting a new swimming lifestyle, you will actually lose some fat.

Published data from as far back as 1983 categorized the body composition (fat mass vs. fat free mass) of athletes in different sports[1]. Swimmers are right in the middle of the rankings (men 12.4%, women 19.5%), and are much leaner than the average college students (men 15%, women 25%). The leanest athletes were found to be those who needed to be powerful and light, such as track and field athletes, (particularly high jumpers) sprinters, and distance runners, and athletes who are categorized into weight classes (boxers, and wrestlers). There appears to be a natural selection pressure at play. People who are inherently leaner have a competitive disadvantage in swimming as they are less buoyant than those with a little more fat. The flip side of the coin is that a person with extra fat (or muscle) is unlikely to excel at the elite level in a sport like high-jump. So, at the level of national and international athletics, it's not the sport that makes the athlete lean or bulky, it is the person who chooses the sport in which they will have best chance to succeed.

To answer the question of whether or not swimmers store more fat than do runners, one study[2] tested a group of elite swimmers, runners, and triathletes during a 45-minute workout at 75% VO_{2max}. The runners and swimmers were tested in their native discipline and the triathletes did both tests. After each exercise session, the athletes were monitored for the total number of calories burned and amount of fat and glucose that they metabolized during a two-hour recovery period.

Although, both the swimmers and runners burned about the same number of calories during the recovery period, there was a clear difference in the types of fuels that were used. The swimmers metabolized significantly more fat than did the runners. Adding to this was the fact that the triathletes showed a clear trend to burning more fat than glucose after their swim sessions than they did during the post-run recovery. The apparent mechanism was an increased use of stored glucose during the swim, perhaps to help keep the body warm. Thus, after 45-minutes of moderately high intensity exercise, the swimmers (and triathletes) had to switch to burning fat during recovery, while the runners still had glucose stores available. So, think about that for a second, not only does this show that swimming does not make you pack on extra weight, but it also reveals the exact opposite, exercise in an aquatic environment makes you burn through your glucose faster so that you have to switch to using fat during recovery.

A subsequent study built on this idea by seeing how swimming in water at different temperatures (68°F, 78.8°F, and 89.6°F) impacted the hormones responsible for stimulating metabolism (thyroid hormones), and the stress hormone (cortisol)[3]. Compared to baseline levels, thyroid hormone was only elevated at 68°F. Elevated thyroid hormones stimulate the burning of extra glucose and fat in order to maintain body temperature. By contrast, swimming at 78.8°F and 89.6°F significantly increased cortisol levels, which reduces fat metabolism and stimulates the breakdown of proteins, not what anyone wants. Clearly, the temperature of the water is of great importance if one of the goals of your new swimming lifestyle is weight loss. Swim in the coldest water you can find and comfortably tolerate.

SWIMMING AND APPETITE

Now, we have come full circle, back to the original question that I asked myself in 2003 when I started training for triathlon, "Does swimming increase appetite more than running or cycling?" It's one thing to do an uncontrolled experiment on yourself outside the strict confines of a laboratory. It's another thing altogether to test that theory in a well-designed, controlled, clinical experiment. Two recent studies have helped to clarify the answer.

In the first study, eleven untrained men were recruited to participate in three trials; one resting control on land, and two exercise trials on a stationary bike modified to be used in the water[4]. The two exercise trials were conducted in warm (91.4°F) and cold (68°F) water. The subjects sat in water up to their chest and rode for 45 minutes at 60% of their VO_{2max} and then recovered for 20-minutes on dry land. For the next hour they were allowed to eat as much food as they wanted from a buffet. Although the subjects didn't expend any more energy during the exercise in the cold water then they did in the warm water, they consumed a whopping 44% more calories during the recovery period after exercise in the cold water than they did after exercise in the warm water.

As a matter of fact, the number of calories consumed after the resting control condition, during which they just sat comfortably in a chair on dry land, was almost the same as they ate after exercise in the warm water. Clearly, exercise in warmer water, just like running and cycling on a hot, humid day, suppresses appetite after exercise, while exercise in cold water makes you hungrier. Now, the 44% increase was probably inflated by the fact that the subjects were given a large variety of foods to choose from, and research shows that when people are given a buffet to choose from, they feel compelled to gorge[5,6].

A more recent study controlled for the overeating impulse by offering an unlimited amount of one kind of food instead of a buffet. A group of aerobically fit men and women exercised for an hour at what they deemed a "hard" intensity, once on a stationary bike, and again during a swimming workout[7]. The exercise sessions were designed to burn the same number of calories. The subjects were then allowed to eat as much of their one food of choice as they wanted during a 90-minute recovery period. As they ate, they answered two questionnaires about their appetite, hunger, and satiety (sense of fullness).

After the swimming session, the subjects consumed 6% more calories than they did after the cycling session. This is less than what I experienced after swimming in my 77°F "normal" pool. Interestingly there was no difference in appetite, hunger, or feelings of fullness between either exercise condition, or the resting control condition. This may be explained by the fact that the pool temperature was somewhat warm at 82.4°F, and the exercise intensity was self-prescribed by perceived exertion instead of being externally controlled. But the important point is that the data is much closer to what I observed in my own behavior than the 44% increase reported after the buffet recovery. Take home message? Have a post-workout snack ready to go, and don't go to a buffet-style restaurant after your workouts. Actually, it's probably good advice to *never* go to a buffet-style restaurant if you're trying to lose weight.

When we zoom out and look at this through a more holistic lens, we can see three key points emerge:

1. Swimming, in and of itself, does not lead to weight gain. If anything, new swimmers should experience some weight loss, provided they follow a reasonable dietary plan.

2. Water temperature matters! In order to extend your swim session and be able to maintain higher intensities, you want to swim in cooler water. But you don't want the water to be too cold or it may stimulate your appetite more than you want, especially if you are trying to lose weight. To be clear, this same thing will happen if you run or cycle in the cold with little insulation. You just notice it after swimming because you transfer more heat, more quickly in water then you do in air.

3. Pay attention to how much you eat after you exercise, and make sure that you don't reward feed. Everyone has done this after a hard workout. You say to yourself, "I'm so proud of myself for finishing that killer set that I am going to eat dinner and dessert and have two beers too." You just consumed twice as many calories as you burned during your workout. This is a lifestyle change, and exercise is never enough. Diet always trumps exercise. Remember that!

CHAPTER 6

Swimming as a Treatment for Neurological Disorders

The year before I met my wife, she was diagnosed with Multiple Sclerosis (MS), a progressive autoimmune disorder that results in her immune system attacking the cells of her brain and spinal cord, the two parts of the central nervous system (CNS). The CNS is the control center for the entire body. It's like the processor in a smart phone. In order for the processor to direct the different parts of your phone to function, it sends electrical impulses along wires, and receives information back to be processed. So, when you tap on the screen, a signal is sent to the processor, telling it that you have activated the phone. The processor responds by instructing the screen to light up so you can use the phone.

The same basic process happens in our bodies anytime we receive information from our external environment and respond to it. For example, as you're walking out of your house you take a misstep and lose your balance for a fraction of a second. That slip is detected by a number of different receptors. Your inner ear detects the rapid shift in your head position, and mechanoreceptors in your muscles that detect stretch, fire as your body begins to fall. The CNS gathers all of this information, processes it, and sends instructions to the appropriate muscles to contract rapidly, allowing you to regain your balance and prevent a tumble.

The speed with which these signals are sent is critically important, a delay, or interruption in the signal can lead to injury. In order to maintain signal integrity and speed, the wires of our CNS (neurons) are wrapped in a coating called myelin that acts like the plastic insulation on the wires that are plugged into your wall outlets right now. The immune systems of MS patients attack the myelin, degrading the insulation. This leads to slower signal transmission, or even a total loss of the signal. People with MS suffer from muscle weakness, depression, vision impairment, and severe fatigue, particularly in heat.

When my wife started experiencing symptoms, I was in the middle of a post-doctoral fellowship in immunology. Of course, I started compiling a library of research on the treatment of MS. Once she began her first immunosuppressant drug therapy, I wanted to know what else we could do to keep her healthy and happy. In my research there were two consistent themes to the successful treatment of MS beyond traditional medical therapies: diet and exercise.

This was right in my wheelhouse. I know how to make healthy food, and keeping her fit was easy as she was an athlete before we met. My wife is not a swimmer. She came from a running background and prefers lacing up her tennies to diving into the deep end. But running in Texas is—for nine months of the year, at least—a hot, humid experience, and there are times when the heat stress is just too much for her. On those days, I take her to the pool to do some light swimming and weighted, water-running. She always feels much better after leaving the pool, especially during a flair. Her anxiety decreases, her thoughts become clearer, and her fatigue is replaced by a state of relaxation and tranquility.

With this first experience under my belt, I started to investigate how swimming impacts three other neurological disorders, Parkinson's disease (PD), cerebral palsy (CP), and autism. My interest in these specific disorders was because I know two people with PD, and two couples with children who suffered from CP and autism respectively. In all four cases, swimming was part of their treatment plan, and by all accounts, improved their health and well-being much more than did traditional medical or therapeutic treatments alone.

SWIMMING AND MULTIPLE SCLEROSIS

A 2012 study examined the effects of an eight-week water-aerobics treatment on the symptoms of MS compared to a control group who maintained their normal treatment[1]. The treatment group exercised for 60-minutes, three times a week, at 50–75% of their maximal heart rate. The outcome measures included subjective measures of fatigue and overall health. There were no differences in any measures between the water-aerobics and control groups at baseline. However, after the eight-week training program the water-aerobics group experienced significant improvements in overall, physical, psychosocial, and cognitive fatigue. They also reported that their energy levels increased, bodily pain decreased, and they perceived fewer limitations, both physical and emotional. By contrast, the control group experienced significant increases in overall and physical fatigue, and no changes in any of the other parameters while on their normal treatment plan.

Ai-Chi, a water-based form of Tai Chi developed in Japan in the early 1990's, is another water-based exercise that improves symptoms of MS[2]. In this case, the control group performed the exact same movements as the Ai-Chi group, but while lying on a yoga mat on dry land. The intervention period lasted twenty-weeks, with follow-up measures taken at four and ten weeks after the intervention ended. Both groups participated in two sessions per week for an hour. In this study, the two primary outcome measures were pain and the frequency and severity of muscle spasms. General fatigue was the secondary measure. Prior to the intervention, there were no differences in any measures of pain, spasm, or fatigue between the Ai-Chi and control groups. While the control group experienced no changes in their symptoms during the 20-week intervention, the Ai-Chi group experienced significant reductions in all outcome measures after the intervention. The relief of symptoms lasted for at least four weeks after the intervention, but most of them returned by 10 weeks.

Whether in healthy people or those with MS, muscle spasms are related to heat stress. As we have discussed, we can dissipate heat much faster during exercise in water than we can while exercising on land. This reduces the incidence of cramps, allowing for exercise to continue for longer, and at higher intensities. Another symptom of MS is generalized muscle weakness, making it difficult to maintain posture during land-based exercise. This is the reason that the control group did Tai Chi while lying, supine on a yoga mat. But this limitation also reduces the quality and duration of the workout.

The buoyant properties of water supported the subjects in the Ai-Chi group, reducing the energy cost of staying upright during the exercise. Finally, the hydrostatic pressure of water increased venous return of blood from the legs to the heart, increasing cardiac output to the muscles, and the brain. All these factors are at play when people with MS swim or exercise in the water.

SWIMMING AND PARKINSON'S DISEASE

Parkinson's Disease (PD) is a degenerative neurological disorder that results in the death of cells that make a neurotransmitter called dopamine.

The symptoms of PD are variable, but most often include muscle weakness, stiffness, tremors, and loss of balance. The part of the brain that is impacted by reduced dopamine levels is called the basal ganglia. It sounds complicated, but in its simplest form, the basal ganglia fine-tunes our movements. Let's say that you want to kick a soccer ball to your daughter who is standing about ten feet from you. That would require less force than kicking the ball to her when she is standing 50 feet away from you. The basal ganglia works together with the part of the brain that tells the leg muscles to kick (the motor cortex) to send the perfect instructions to the leg muscles. Without dopamine, these instructions may not be sent correctly, often there is not enough force generation for large, powerful movements, and this presents as muscle weakness.

On the other end of the spectrum, dopamine allows the basal ganglia to inhibit other movements that we *don't* want to happen. As you are holding this book in your hands, your motor cortex is telling your arms to hold your hands still in front of you so you can read the words on the page. This is a very complex set of instructions that involves thousands of neurons and muscle fibers. Without a healthy basal ganglia, you may experience uncontrolled contractions in the hands and arms, called tremors. To put this into context, you can look at videos of Michael J. Fox from the time of his diagnosis in 1991 and contrast them to how he looks today. Despite the best treatments in the world, he suffers from noticeable tremors and stiffness, particularly in his arms and face. Interestingly, while researching this topic, I found my way to the Michael J. Fox Foundation webpage where I discovered an article titled, "Swimming Away Parkinson's." It's a good read.

Physical therapy treatments for PD focus on improving muscle function, in particular strength, flexibility, and fitness, in order to restore and maintain balance, reducing the risk of falls. The muscles that help us maintain balance are called postural muscles. Examples include the calf muscles, hamstrings, pectorals, and the latissimus dorsi (big, upper back muscles).

When the center of mass shifts away from a central, resting position, the postural muscles are directed to quickly contract, bringing the body back to a balanced posture. Parkinson's disease weakens these muscles, making them respond more slowly, or with less force, increasing the risk of falls. As with any kind of exercise, the best way to improve the function of postural muscles when we are off balance is to intentionally make us lose our balance, in a controlled setting that reduces the risk of injury. The simplest example is to have someone stand with their feet side by side and reach out with one arm to grab an object in front of them. For healthy people, they won't even notice a change in balance as the arm is moved from away from the center of mass, but for someone with PD, this subtle shift in weight can cause a major loss of balance.

The most commonly used measure of balance is the Berg Balance Scale (BBS), a questionnaire that ranks 14 actions related to functional balance from 0-4. A cumulative score between 0-20 means the subject is wheelchair bound. A score of 21-40 means they can walk with assistance, and 41-56 means they are independent. A study from Italy randomly assigned PD patients to one of two groups, a control group that performed 60 minutes of cardiovascular and strength training (including flexibility, strength, and balance exercises) on dry land, or an experimental group that performed the same exercises in water up to the level of the sternum (mid-chest)[3].

Subjects exercised five days a week for two months. As expected, there were no differences between the groups before the intervention. After the two months of treatment, scores on the BBS improved more for the hydrotherapy group (41.3 to 51.2) than for the control group (43.9 to 49.9). The most important improvement observed was an 80% reduction in the number of falls reported in the hydrotherapy group when compared to the control group (19% fewer falls), a fourfold difference between the two conditions.

Similar to the effects of swimming on MS patients, exercise in an aquatic environment provides additional benefits that land-based exercises do not. The buoyant properties of water and hydrostatic pressure prop up the body during exercise, reducing the stress on the postural muscles. This delays fatigue, allowing the subjects to exercise at higher intensities for longer durations. Since water is more viscous than air, there is more resistance to movement, making the muscles stronger. But the most important element of exercising in water is the reduced risk of falls. The subjects in the hydrotherapy group reported feeling safer and more confident during the exercise sessions than did their land-based counterparts.

SWIMMING AS A TREATMENT FOR CEREBRAL PALSY

Cerebral palsy (CP) is the most common motor disability in children and typically results in lifelong motor impairment. Physical therapy focuses on improving, or maintaining walking, as this is the most important skill required for keeping up with their healthy peers during childhood development. Unfortunately, CP makes exercise difficult because the muscles are often weak, and spasms are common. Another frequent symptom of CP is generalized muscle pain that increases in severity during exercise, limiting the intensity and duration of activity. Recently, swimming has been shown to be a safe and effective means of increasing muscle strength, and endurance, without increasing pain.

Children with CP were randomly assigned to either a swimming group or a control group[4]. The swimming group received supervised swim lessons for 40-50 minutes per session, twice a week for ten weeks. Both groups maintained their normal physical therapy schedules. The primary outcome measure was the distance that they could walk in one minute. Each group was assessed before and after the ten-week intervention and five weeks after the intervention. The control group was then invited to participate in the same swimming lessons.

The swimming group walked a further 11.6 meters after the swimming intervention and this increased to 18.9 meters at the five-week follow-up. By contrast, the distance covered by the control group after the intervention actually decreased by 7.6 meters. Neither group reported any changes in generalized pain for the course of the treatment period. These results show that swimming is a safe and effective means of increasing muscle strength and cardiovascular endurance in children with CP, without causing pain or muscle spasm. Best of all, the improvements in health translate to functional land-based activities, i.e., walking.

SWIMMING AS A TREATMENT FOR AUTISM SPECTRUM DISORDER

Autism Spectrum Disorder (ASD) is a neurodevelopmental disorder that impacts the social, behavioral, and sometimes, physical development of children. People with ASD often struggle with processing instructions and verbal communication. Many people with ASD also struggle with how they respond to physical stimuli. Visual, audio, and physical stimuli that you and I would not even notice, can overwhelm the senses of some people with ASD. The flip side of the coin is lack of sensation that can often occur, leading to characteristic behaviors that are thought to be an attempt to try to feel something. These include repetitive rocking, tapping, moaning, and hitting oneself. As a direct result of these actions, or perhaps out of frustration, people with ASD often suffer from mental health issues including anxiety and depression, and behavioral problems including antisocial and aggressive behaviors.

Two recent studies have shown that aquatic exercise significantly improved symptoms of anxiety, depression, and behavioral problems in children with ASD, and these effects lasted for 8-10 weeks after the swimming intervention[5, 6]. But, in reading these studies, it was clear that neither group of investigators had a good explanation for how swimming improves symptoms of ASD. So, I set out to do some more research of my own. Before I got very far, I happened across a movie about a person whom I had never heard of before, Temple Grandin. The movie, eponymously named, is great, and I highly recommend it.

Temple Grandin is a scientist and engineer in livestock management, creating more humane ways of herding and slaughtering animals. She also happens to have ASD. As a small child she often felt the urge for deep pressure stimulation, but being hugged, or even held, was overwhelming. When visiting her aunt's farm as a child she watched calves being put into a vaccination chute, a device that clamps on either side of a calf, holding it still while it is vaccinated. Temple observed that although the calves were agitated when entering the chute, they almost immediately calmed when being squeezed.

In college she made a prototype for herself that she called a hug-box, or squeezebox. She would lay on her stomach in the V-shaped device and pulled a handle that would move the walls of the V together, applying a controlled, deep squeeze. This calmed her hypersensitivity. My theory is that the hydrostatic pressure of water applies a gentle, constant pressure that provides a calming effect to those with ASD. This proposed mechanism is supported by findings that older children with more moderate forms of ASD experience improved sleep after an eight-week swim intervention[5].

The benefits of swimming and aquatic exercise in the treatment of these four neurological disorders reveal some universal mechanisms that can benefit otherwise healthy people.

- Buoyancy supports the body, reducing the energy requirement for maintaining posture.

- Hydrostatic pressure increases venous return of blood to the heart, improving Q, reducing the strain on the heart.

- Heat stress is reduced, and water conducts heat transfer from the body faster than air.

- All these factors increase the duration and intensity of exercise, precisely what is needed to improve physical fitness, and quality of life.

CHAPTER 7

Swimming for Pain Management

Imagine holding the metal handle of a pot that you just put on the stove. After a minute or two, you can feel that the handle is now warm, and it is slowly getting hot. Before you burn yourself, you feel the sensation of pain in your skin.

Pain is a mechanism that signals the presence of damaged tissue, or that continuing a particular behavior may lead to damaged tissue. Another example of pain signaling that is more specific to exercise is called delayed onset muscle soreness (DOMS). Let's say It's been a busy few weeks and you haven't had time to get to the gym. On your first day back, instead of taking it easy, you decide to pick up where you left off six weeks ago and do three sets of ten squats at 80% of your maximum, a very high-intensity workout. During your workout your leg and gluteus muscles develop tiny tears that will need repair. You don't feel much that night, but when you wake up the next morning your legs feel stiff and sore. As you go to sit down at the dining room table for coffee, you feel the sharp pain of DOMS.

In both cases the signals of pain being sent to the brain are coming from pain receptors called nociceptors. We have different kinds of nociceptors that respond to different stimuli. The hot pot handle was detected by thermoreceptors. Delayed onset muscle soreness is caused by inflammation. As white blood cells swoop into the muscles to clear out the damaged tissue, they release several chemicals that are detected by chemoreceptors, sensitizing them to send signals that are translated by our brain as a dull ache. But, when we press on the muscles or make them contract, mechanoreceptors in the muscles send additional signals to the brain, saying, "Hey! Stop moving this muscle, it's hurt!"

Here, we're going to focus on mechanoreceptors, as these are the most common communicators of pain, both acute and chronic, when it comes to musculoskeletal damage. We have evolved the ability to tune out our mechanoreceptors when the stimulation lasts too long. For example, when you pull your shirt over your head, you immediately feel the fabric against your skin. You can feel its texture, whether it is rough or soft, sleek or heavy. But in short order you don't feel it anymore, at least at the level that you are consciously aware of it. This is what you want to happen. If you had a constant stream of information flooding your brain saying, "You're wearing a shirt! You're wearing a shirt!" you would be in sensory overload almost immediately. In this example, we want our mechanoreceptors to warn us when something is on our skin that is not *supposed* to be there and may be dangerous. Although you don't want to feel your shirt, you *do* want to feel the fire ant climbing up your leg.

We can use this desensitizing mechanism to reduce our perception of pain. Think about what you did the last time that you stubbed your toe or struck your "funny bone." You probably grabbed your toe and squeezed it, or you rubbed your elbow really hard. The external pressure desensitized the nociceptors that were triggered and inhibited them from sending as many pain signals as possible to the brain. We can do the same thing with chronic pain. Many people with arthritic joints wear garments that compress the surrounding tissues, reducing the sensation of pain.

Humans have understood that swimming, or just being immersed in water reduces pain for as long as we've been wading into rivers and lakes. But the research on the mechanism of how this process works is quite new, and most of the studies that exist have been conducted in animals. Four probable mechanisms of action have been identified:

1. The hydrostatic pressure of water compresses the mechanorecep-tors of the skin and muscles, inhibiting them from signaling pain.

2. As we swim, water constantly flows over the skin. Just like wearing a shirt, the mechanoreceptors in the skin quickly become desensitized to the movement of the water over its surface. This also reduces their transmission of pain and discomfort signals.

3. The buoyancy of water lifts the body off the ground, decompress-ing the joints, particularly the feet, knees, hips, and vertebrae of the lower back. Unloading sore muscles and joints reduces signals of pain.

4. Swimming reduces inflammation, and by extension, the sensitiv-ity of nociceptors to detecting pain[1].

Although land-based exercise is also associated with pain reduction in the long term, these four elements of swimming and water-based exercise are unique to an aquatic environment.

The newest areas of research are focused on how swimming effects the production of natural painkillers that we make in our brain, partic-ularly during exercise. Endorphins and enkephalins bind to the same receptors as do opioids, reducing the sensation of pain and improving mood. Endocannabinoids are another group of substances that bind to the same receptors as does the active ingredient in Marijuana. Similar to endorphins and enkephalins, endocannabinoids reduce the sensation of pain, improve mood, reduce anxiety, and increase appetite. Hopefully future studies will be able to clarify how swimming reduces pain so that we can better utilize this simple treatment. In the meantime, when you need some relief from your nagging aches or more severe pain, go for a swim.

CHAPTER 8

Swimming for Mental Health and Wellness

Over the course of the last decade mental illness has gone from being a diagnosis that was largely misunderstood and kept secret to one championed by world famous actors, athletes, and political figures. Mental health awareness campaigns have brought attention to the prevalence of the issue, nearly 20% of Americans suffer from some form of mental illness, with around 5% suffering from serious mental health issues (according to statistics published by the National Alliance of Mental Illness). But the recent attention paid to the commonality of mental illness has also made it so that those suffering, and their loved ones, don't feel so alone when it comes to discussions about diagnosis and treatment. Although there is no substitute for the proper medical and psychological treatment of mental illness, exercise, particularly swimming has been shown to provide remarkable beneficial effects on both mental and cognitive health.

SWIMMING, ANXIETY AND DEPRESSION

Anxiety disorders are the most commonly diagnosed mental health disorder in the United States. More than 40 million adults, approximately 18% of the population, are diagnosed each year. Nearly half of these people are also diagnosed with chronic depression (according to statistics put forth by the Anxiety and Depression Association of America). Both conditions are highly treatable with counseling, medications, and exercise. On this last note, swimming has been shown to be an extremely effective treatment for symptoms of anxiety and depression.

Self-reported levels of general mental health, anxiety, and depression were measured in two groups of men between the ages of 45-55 years[1]. The subjects were split into a control group that did not exercise, and an experimental group that participated in water jogging for 30 minutes at 60–70% of maximal heart rate, three times a week, for eight weeks. Questionnaire data about general health was collected before and after the eight-week trial.

There were no differences in any of the measures of mental health between the groups before the study began. The control group experienced no changes in any measurement during the study. However, after the eight-weeks of water jogging, the exercise group showed significant improvements in their symptoms of general mental health disorder (12%), anxiety (11.5%), and depression (20%).

Similar benefits were observed in a case study on the effects of open-water swimming on the symptoms of major depressive disorder (MDD) in a 24-year old woman who was eight months post-partum[2]. The patient in question was originally diagnosed when she was 17 but had shown signs of depression since her early teen years. These included anger, anxiety, dark mood, and self-harm. Antidepressants and counseling therapy had not been effective. Before beginning the open-water swimming intervention, the subject had expressed that she wanted to be symptom-free and wanted to stop taking her medications because they made her feel as though she was in a "chemical fog", a complaint common of both antidepressant and anxiolytic drugs.

She began a supervised program of open-water swimming with a swim instructor, once or twice a week, eventually extending her swims to 30-minutes in duration. After four months of swimming, she no longer needed medication, and this was still the case after a one-year follow up. Clearly, additional evidence is needed before swimming, particularly cold, open-water swimming can be prescribed as a treatment for mental illness, but these two reports are promising. But similar results have been reported after participation in land-based forms of exercise, both aerobic and anaerobic, e.g., resistance training. So, although the previous two studies are interesting, they don't provide any evidence that being in an aquatic environment, separate from exercise, is of particular benefit. That is where the following studies about floating come in.

Floatation-REST (Restricted Environmental Stimulation Technique) is a method of sensory deprivation during which subjects float in a quiet, dark, pod filled with warm, salty water that makes you more buoyant. Floatation-REST has recently been used as an experimental treatment for anxiety[3]. In this experiment the subjects were recruited from an outpatient psychiatric care facility, and randomly assigned to either the experimental group that participated in twelve, 45-minute floatation sessions over seven weeks, or a control group that did not (although they continued to receive their normal treatments).

All subjects had a prolonged history of anxiety. Measurements of sleep quality, depression, anxiety, and the ability to regulate emotions were taken in both groups before the trial started, after four weeks of treatment, and after the last session. The floatation group participated in a follow up interview at six months after the intervention concluded.

As would be expected, there were no differences between the two groups in any of the mental health measures before the intervention and the control group showed no changes over the seven weeks. But the floatation group experienced significant improvements in sleep quality, depression, anxiety, and their ability to regulate their emotional state. These improvements began at four weeks of treatment and were larger still by the seventh week. Most impressive was the fact that these improvements were largely maintained over the six months following the floatation-REST intervention. Of equal importance was the reduction in the use of medications over the seven weeks of floatation therapy: antidepressant use decreased by 20%, anxiolytics decreased by 17%, and the proportion of subjects taking sleeping aids went from 12% to 0%. These changes were also well maintained at the six-month follow-up.

Building on these results, a study conducted at the Laureate Institute for Brain Research, Tulsa, Oklahoma, measured the impacts of a single, 60-minute, floatation-REST session on a battery of measures of mental health and wellbeing, including anxiety, depression, stress, serenity, and overall well-being in a group of patients suffering from chronic anxiety and depression (experimental group), and a reference control group of people who did not suffer from any form of mental illness[4]. Unlike the previous study, in this case, both groups were treated with a single floatation-REST session.

Not surprisingly, the experimental group had much higher scores for general anxiety before the floatation session than did the control group. Although both groups experienced less anxiety after the session, the experimental group saw a huge drop to levels similar to those of their non-anxious counterparts. The anxious group experienced statistically significant drops in self-reported levels of pain, fatigue, sleepiness, depression, and muscle tension, while the positive outcomes of feeling refreshed, serene, relaxed, and happy were significantly increased.

Now, in science, the critical threshold of when an experiment "works" is when we reach a level of statistical significance. This means that we are at least 95% certain that the changes observed in mood are because of the floatation-REST treatment, and not because of random chance. But just because floatation-REST has an effect doesn't mean that the effect is very impressive. We see this often in weight-loss studies. For example, when explaining this concept to my students I like to cite a study on the use of green coffee bean extract for weight loss in otherwise healthy, over-weight people. The group that received the supplement for four weeks lost significantly more weight (approximately 5.8 pounds) than did the control group (no change). But this represents a change of only 3.5% of their initial body weight. They very likely could have accomplished more with diet and exercise[5].

In order to see what the true impact of a treatment is, we need to use an additional measure called an effect size. As a reference point, a large effect size is 0.8 or greater. The effect size of the weight loss that occurred after consuming green coffee bean extract was 0.4, or moderate in size. In all, 14 measures of mental health improved after floatation, and all had effect sizes greater than 0.8. The three largest were increased feelings of serenity (2.11), reduced anxiety (2.15), and a feeling of being refreshed (2.39). An equivalent effect size in the green coffee bean extract study would be a weight loss of almost 22%, or 36 pounds! The point I'm making is that the magnitude of the improvements in mental health observed by the Laureate Institute are rarely seen in human studies. These results show that just being in water can greatly benefit your mental health. When you add the additional benefits that come with aerobic exercise, you quickly see why swimming is truly the best prescription for a healthy lifestyle.

So, let's review what we have learned. Aerobic training in an aquatic environment in the form of water jogging or swimming improves mea-sures of mental health. Although the additional benefits of exercise are obvious, there is clear evidence that just floating in water, in combination with sensory deprivation dramatically improves mood and decreases symptoms of anxiety and depression. Incredibly, there is published data that shows that the mere presence of a pool in your neighborhood can improve the mental health and well-being of the surrounding community. Conversely, the results from a study in Glasgow, Scotland, UK show when a pool is shut down, there is a rapid, and measurable decline in the mood of the population[6].

In one neighborhood, Riverside, a community center that included a pool opened in January 2000. In the second neighborhood, Parkview, the local council closed their facility in December 1999. Only long-term residents, defined as having lived in the neighborhoods for at least four years, were included in the respective focus groups. All surveys occurred 14–18 months after the opening or closure of the respective facility.

Interestingly, although both communities spoke about how the pool was important as a place to get exercise, most residents rarely used it for that purpose. Instead, the pool was a place to make connections with their neighbors and friends. Most respondents reported that they went to the pool to wade and relax with friends and family. Although there were other publicly available areas to exercise, including parks and soccer fields, the residents did not use those facilities as common gathering areas. It appears that a community pool is the human equivalent of a watering hole, a place to commune and relax.

Swimming and Cognitive Function

Cognitive function is an umbrella term that includes several mental abilities including learning, thinking, reasoning, memory recall, problem solving, attention, and decision-making. It is well established that aerobic exercise, either in terms of a single bout, or long-term training, improves cognitive function by increasing blood flow to the brain. As exercise intensity increases, the heart delivers more blood to all active tissues, namely the muscles, skin, and brain. But the primary stimulus that increases blood flow to the brain specifically is the increased circulating levels of CO_2 in blood.

The brain is very sensitive to changes in the ratio of O_2 to CO_2. If CO_2 increases or O_2 decreases even slightly, the cardiorespiratory systems are directed to increase blood flow to the brain to maintain the desired proportions. In addition to removing the extra CO_2 produced during exercise, the additional blood delivers more O_2 and several growth factors that promote brain health and improve cognitive function.

When we move exercise to the water, both cardiac output and circulating levels of CO_2 are increased when compared to land-based aerobic exercise. The hydrostatic pressure of water immersion alone shifts blood volume from the legs toward to the heart, increasing cardiac output, and the volume of blood available to flow through the brain[7, 8]. More importantly, during swimming, we hold our breath for short periods of time, resulting in even higher levels of CO_2 in the blood than we experience during land-based exercise.

A single 20-minute session of moderately paced breaststroke has been shown to improve cognitive function. The test subjects included a group of runners, and another of swimmers[9]. Subjects were shown a red or green dot positioned on the left or right side respectively, of a computer screen. Using two clickers, one in each hand, the subjects were instructed to press the corresponding button as quickly as possible. In reaction tests, both accuracy and speed are equally important. It's great if you always click the correct button, but if it takes you a long time to do it, your reaction time is pretty poor. By the same token, if you always get the answer wrong, it doesn't matter how fast you do it. Accordingly, the test was scored as the ratio between the reaction time and the error rate, so the lower the number, the faster, and more accurate the performance.

There was no difference between the groups at any point during the experiment, but when all subjects were combined into one group, the reaction time test scores were significantly improved after the swimming session. As expected, swimming led to significant increases in cardiac output, circulating CO_2 levels, and brain blood flow.

Although the precise mechanism by which swimming improves mental health remains to be fully understood I have a theory that is supported by the science. Think about all the physiological changes that occur when you step into a pool of water. Buoyancy gently lifts you off the ground, unloading your tired muscles and bones, cradling you as you float. The hydrostatic pressure of water applies a gentle hug, pushing fluids from your swollen limbs back into circulation, easing the load on your heart and shifting blood flow to your brain. Both properties stimulate the part of your nervous system that controls relaxation. To me, this description of water as a safe place, a harbor in the storm of everyday life, sounds like when we floated in amniotic fluid during embryological development. Think about it, in a very real sense, we all came from the water. All of us spent nine months immersed in water in the safest place that nature ever conceived, our mothers' womb. Perhaps swimming provides the environmental cues necessary for your body to do a factory reset as it were, bringing us back to the state of being where we all began, cradled, safe and warm in our mother's arms.

PART 2

SWIMMING AS A LIFESTYLE

CHAPTER 9

Getting Started

You now have a working understanding of the wide range of health benefits that swimming can provide. Now, you need to determine not only what your goals are, but how best to achieve them. Are you interested in swimming for the health benefits only? Do you want to swim by yourself on your schedule, or do you want to join a club? Are you interested in competing in Masters, or open water swimming? The answers to these questions will likely be a moving target, changing as your swimming skills improve, or over the course of any given season. There are benefits and drawbacks to each approach, and we'll go over each in this chapter.

MASTERS OR SOLO SWIMMING?

After graduating from college, I took a long hiatus from swimming. This ended when I started competing in triathlon. Since I had been a very successful swimming coach for several years, I thought that I could train myself without issue, and I was right in terms of the logistics of writing workouts and doing the swimming. But, in short order I could feel that my swimming performances were plateauing. I needed to swim with other people, and I needed someone else to be in charge of writing my workouts if I was going to get faster.

Luckily, I was good friends with the head swimming coach at the University of Houston, where I was doing my doctoral studies. He invited me to swim with his club team. Although most of the people in the pool were teenagers, there were about 10 to 12 regular Masters swimmers like myself. I knew I had made the right decision during our first practice. It wasn't that the workouts were better or tougher, but having other people around me brought out my competitive spirit and I swam much harder.

The other positive aspect about being on a team was that people held me accountable for showing up to practice *and* for swimming hard while at practice. A cumulative effect happens with this element of team swimming. Our Masters swimmers: men and women, younger and older, were all quite capable of keeping up with the high school and college-age members of the team. This led us to some very intense workouts where we were all racing each other, cheering each other on, sometimes doing a little friendly trash-talking, but always swimming hard. By my first race of the season, the impact of these workouts was evident. I won the race by over five minutes, and it started with a dominant open water swim. For the remainder of my triathlon career, I stuck with Masters swimming.

In this particular scenario, we had a smaller group of Masters swimmers who were crashing the club kids' party, as it were. But these kinds of workouts aren't for everyone, and our coach had another practice session that was just for Masters swimmers, no youngster allowed. Some of these members raced, but most of these folks were there to maintain their fitness or to learn how to improve their stroke technique. I had the privilege to be the stand-in coach for this group on several occasions. Although the vibe in these practice sessions was much more laid back than ours, the camaraderie was still readily apparent. If someone was absent from practice, everyone knew it, and if there was a concern, inevitably that person would get a phone call, checking on them, and asking them to come back to the pool soon.

Obviously, all teams are different, but I would wager that most Masters programs have this kind of dynamic. If you think this is what is going to motivate you to get to practice and stick with swimming, then I encourage you to find the nearest team and give it a try. My only word of caution is to be patient when it comes to finding your place in the team. Many Masters swimmers have been together for a long time. When I joined, it took me about a month to really feel at home.

If being on a team is not for you, or it simply does not fit into your schedule, the other option is to find a coach who will write your workouts and track your progress remotely. This requires a little more legwork on your part because you will have to track some data and report it back to your coach. But the advantage of this option is that your coach can be anywhere on the planet. This method works best for more independent athletes who are data driven, but if you know that you're going to struggle with reporting your data, this method will limit your success, because your coach won't know if the workout was too easy, or too hard. So, before making a final decision and spending money on an online coach (who can be pretty pricey), take all of these factors into consideration.

THE BENEFITS OF COMPETITION

Competitive swimming for adults can take many forms. There are Masters swimming meets that range from local meets, to state, national, and even world championships. In my part of the country, open water swimming is just starting to gain a foothold, but there are regularly scheduled open water swimming competitions all over the country. Of course, swimming is the first of the three disciplines in a triathlon, a very popular sport for first time competitors.

Depending on the competition in question, it can take anywhere from a month (Masters swim meet) to six months (sprint triathlon) to get someone ready to safely, and competently compete. In most of these cases, the sense of accomplishment that comes with completing their first race is enough to get them to register for another event. This is why I push competition. No matter your innate motivation during a competition, the end results will always be the same, i.e., you will stick with the program, and you will work harder. The combination of those two outcomes is that you will experience greater health benefits than if you did not compete.

Now, this is not to say that you can't improve your health with exercise alone, of course you can. The point is that most people derive *more* health benefits from training for a specific competitive event. The added health benefits are beyond improving cardiovascular function and bone mineral density. Competition improves mental health by making you part of a community. Competition gives you purpose. In short, competition is a microcosm of life. We strive to improve ourselves and grow every day.

HIIT AND SWIMMING

My triathlon club in Houston was a volunteer organization. We all helped in any way we could, and since I was completing a PhD in exercise physiology, people often turned to me to ask questions about training. At one of our monthly meetings, I gave a talk on the importance of the pre-race meal. After my presentation, we opened the floor to questions. One question that has always stuck with me was from a person who had volunteered to be a guide swimmer for a blind athlete. I had heard of this in running, but never swimming. He would swim, tethered to, and just in front of the blind athlete, a very cool thing to do, if you ask me. His question was whether or not the slow-paced swimming he was doing during his training sessions as a guide would impact his performance in the future. My answer was simple; long, slow swimming produces long, slow swimmers. The solution was to add a few, shorter-distance, sprint sets to maintain his speed.

This brings us to the idea of High-Intensity Interval Training (HIIT). HIIT is not a new training technique, but it has been popularized in mainstream media over the last 10 to 15 years. The point of HIIT is to train at the highest intensity possible for the longest, total duration. High intensity is defined as anything above 80% of your maximal aerobic intensity, which you can gauge with a heart rate monitor. Research has clearly shown that HIIT provides greater health benefits than traditional endurance training (i.e., between 50–70% intensity). But the best part is that a HIIT workout can take less than half of the time in the pool to derive the same cardiovascular benefits as does a moderate-intensity, long swim. For those with a tight schedule, HIIT is the way to go.

This was clearly shown in a group of sedentary women with mild hypertension who were randomly assigned to either an endurance swimming (control), or a HIIT swimming group[1]. Both groups trained for 15 weeks with the control group swimming continuously for an hour each session, and the HIIT group completing 6-10, 30-second, all out sprints with a two-minute recovery between each sprint. After the 15 weeks, both groups showed similar improvements in blood pressure, resting heart rate, and total body fat mass.

As expected, the control group did better on the swimming endurance test, and the HIIT group did better in the swimming sprint test. But both groups improved compared to before the 15-week intervention. The biggest take-home message from this study was that although the HIIT group was in the pool for less than half the time of the control group, they got the same health benefits, making for a very efficient workout. We'll talk more about HIIT when we get to the 12-week training plans.

Swimming is a versatile activity that can be done in a pool or a lake, alone or as part of a group activity. Joining a Masters swim team or swimming club provides a level of comradery, accountability, and goal achievement that many find beneficial when starting a new fitness routine. Now, let's shift gears and find out what equipment you will need to get started on your new journey as a swimmer for life.

CHAPTER 10

Learning the Basics

Before you're ready to start any training plan, we need to cover the keys to success when beginning a new aerobic training program: tracking exercise intensity with heart rate and determining how fast you need to swim in order to get fit, faster.

DETERMINING YOUR MAXIMAL SWIMMING HEART RATE

If I were to start training a new client today for a long distance, open water race taking place six months from now, the two key pieces of data that I would want to collect would be her VO_{2max} and lactate threshold (LT). I would put her in flume so that I could control her swimming speed during a graded exercise test. She in turn would wear a mouthpiece attached to a gas analyzer so that I could collect her exhaled air. I would also need to take periodic blood samples. From this data I could determine her aerobic fitness (VO_{2max}) and the swimming speed that she could sustain for a long time before fatiguing, i.e., her LT.

In order to stimulate the physiological adaptations required to make her faster, I would design workouts that would have her swimming right at, or just above, her LT speed. Since the LT is a moving target, as she gets faster, her LT will occur at a higher intensity (faster swimming speed) than it did when she had just started, so we need to take these measures every few weeks. If we don't see improvements in VO_{2max} and LT, we know that we need to change something in the training program.

Since you will not have access to any of the equipment necessary to measure these parameters, we will need to rely on other simpler, cheaper methods. Luckily, we have two that work very well, your heart rate, and self-reported perceived exertion. Heart rate correlates extremely well with exercise intensity. So, if we have an accurate measure of your maximal heart rate, we can very closely estimate your relative intensity during swimming. You can estimate your max heart rate (HR_{max}) by using the equation,

$$HR_{max} = 208 - (0.7 \times \text{Age in years})$$

So, my estimated max heart rate is

$$HR_{max} = 208 - (0.7 \times 47) = 175 \text{ beats per minute}$$

Although this is a good place to start, there is always some error associated with estimating HR_{max}, and this equation was also developed using running as the exercise. Because swimming is done in water (hydrostatic pressure), in the prone position, and requires less muscle mass than running, your swimming max heart rate will be lower than your running max heart. I can tell you that my measured running HR_{max} is 180 bpm while my measured swimming HR_{max} is 173 bpm. So, after you have done a few weeks of light training, I always recommend an easy test to measure your true swimming HR_{max}. If you look at any of the 12-week training programs provided in the back of this book, this test set occurs in the third and eighth week of training. You will need a HR monitor, or preferable a smart watch with both HR monitor and pace clock functions.

After warming up for about 20 minutes of progressively faster swimming, you'll do four sets of four 50-yard swims, with each set getting faster. You'll then finish with a set of two all-out 50-yard sprints. During the first set, take 20 seconds rest between repetitions; during the second set, take 15 seconds, and so on. Between each set, swim for 1:30 at a gentle pace. This is what is called *active recovery*. In other words, swim very slowly, but don't stray too far from the wall because that 1:30 will pass quickly.

SET	REPS	REST BETWEEN REPS	RPE INTENSITY (1–10)
1	4	20 sec	3–4
		1:30 ACTIVE RECOVERY	
2	4	15 sec	5–6
		1:30 ACTIVE RECOVERY	
3	4	10 sec	7
		1:30 ACTIVE RECOVERY	
4	4	5 sec	8–9
		1:30 ACTIVE RECOVERY	
5	2	5 sec	10

Check your HR for about 5–10 seconds after each set of four. Remember the point is to get you to your HR_{max}. We don't want you to recover completely between the swims that come at the end of the workout. Swim as fast as you can for the last two 50s. You should be panting between the two repeats.

Now that you have your HR_{max} you can determine your heart rate training zones. We will break them down by relative intensity into five zones:

- Zone 1: Very Light (50–60%)
- Zone 2: Light (61–70%)
- Zone 3: Moderate (71–80%)/Just below LT
- Zone 4: Hard (81–90%)/Just above LT

- Zone 5: Very Hard (91–100%)

Before you start doing any math, you will also need to measure your resting heart rate ($HR_{resting}$). The best way to measure $HR_{resting}$ is during sleep with your smart watch. If you don't have one, palpate your heart rate at your neck or wrist immediately after you wake up, and before you get out of bed in the morning. Using a watch, count the number of heartbeats that happen in six seconds and multiply that number by ten. My $HR_{resting}$ is 64 bpm, and this represents a 1 on my rating of perceived exertion (RPE) scale. With this data, we need to calculate one more value before we can generate our heart rate training zones; it is called our heart rate reserve (HRR).

$$HRR = HR_{max} - HR_{resting}$$

Still using my example, my HRR is:

$$HRR = 175 - 64 = 111 \text{ BPM}$$

The reason we need to calculate our HRR is because we need to know what range of our heart rate we can actually manipulate. At first glance, it looks like I should have 175 BPM to work with, but my HR can't be any lower than 64 BPM unless I'm dying. The range of HR rate that I can play with is actually 111 BPM, from 64-175 BPM.

Now, let's calculate my Zone 1 range of 50–60%.

- Zone 1: Very Light (50%) = 50% × 111(HRR) + 64($HR_{resting}$) = 120 bpm
- Zone 1: Very Light (60%) = 60% × 111(HRR) + 64($HR_{resting}$) = 131 bpm

In order to stay in the very light range of relative intensities, I need to keep my HR between 120 and 131 bpm. Any value between $HR_{resting}$ and 119 bpm is where I will be when I am walking around and doing my everyday activities that are not intense enough to be considered exercise. You can program these training zones into most smart watches so that they make an audible "beep" if you go too hard or too easy. Follow the same method to determine the remaining training zones just like I have in the table below.

You can use this to see how hard you're really working on any given day, typically during longer swims of 500 yard or more. You will see in the training programs that I have a few longer swims to be done in Zone 1, 2, or 3. Take a periodic check of your heart rate and adjust your speed to raise or lower your heart rate appropriately. In short order you'll be able to do this by feel and won't require frequent checks of your smart watch. One final note, just like your LT, your $HR_{resting}$ will change (decrease) as your fitness improves. That means that you should recalculate your ranges until your $HR_{resting}$ stabilizes. I recommend measuring your $HR_{resting}$ regularly and adjusting accordingly.

TRAINING ZONE DESCRIPTION	HEART RATE RANGE (BPM)
Zone 1: Very Light (50–60%)	120–131
Zone 2: Light (61–70%)	132–142
Zone 3: Moderate (71–80%)	143–153
Zone 4: Hard (81–90%)	154–164
Zone 5: Very Hard (91–100%)	165–175

RATING OF PERCEIVED EXERTION (RPE)

The other method is more subjective. It is called a rating of perceived exertion (RPE). There are a number of methods to determine this, but the easiest was developed by Gunner Borg in the early 1980's and involves rating how hard you feel you are working by pointing to a color that corresponds to your perceived exertion on chart from 1-10 as follows[1]:

- **Dark Blue (1): Very Light Activity.** Hardly any exertion, but more than sleeping or watching TV, etc.

- **Light Blue (2–3): Light Activity.** Feels like you can maintain the effort for hours. Easy to breathe and carry on a conversation.

- **Green (4–6): Moderate Activity.** Breathing heavily. Can hold a short conversation. Still somewhat comfortable but becoming noticeably more challenging.

- **Yellow (7–8): Vigorous Activity.** Borderline uncomfortable. Short of breath, can speak a sentence.

- **Orange (9): Very Hard Activity.** Very difficult to maintain exercise intensity. Can barely breathe and speak only a few words.

- **Red (10): Max Effort Activity.** Feels almost impossible to keep going. Completely out of breath, unable to talk. Cannot maintain for more than a very short time.

DETERMINING YOUR OPTIMAL SWIMMING INTERVALS

Exercising by heart rate and perceived exertion (feel) is a fine way to train, but I prefer to swim at pace, meaning that we set a certain swimming speed that we want you to maintain regardless of what your heart rate is. That said, if you know what you're doing, it's pretty easy to set paces that will keep you within one of the first three training zones. The last two, higher-intensity training zones are accomplished by doing short sets of sprint swimming, well above your VO_{2max} pace, with lots of recovery time between swims. These sets will be clearly marked on your sprint days in the training programs.

Aerobic endurance training is done using one of two methods:

1. Doing one long, and relatively low-intensity swim
2. Breaking up your workout into smaller chunks that you can swim at higher intensities

High-intensity exercise stimulates greater physiological adaptations, cardiovascular, pulmonary, and metabolic, etc., than does long-duration, low-intensity work. These changes happen faster as well. As you will see in the training programs, much of the work is broken up into interval sets. When I coached high school and college swimmers, I knew the intervals that they could handle when they were swimming in Zone 1 for warm-up and cool-down, in Zone 2 to maintain fitness, or in Zone 3, at, or near LT to improve fitness and racing speed. Most coaches will use a combination of the two methods; I'll do the same in the training programs.

Over the course of a competitive season, there is plenty of time to determine who belongs in which lane. However, when you are new to swimming, determining your intervals can be difficult. Because of this, most new swimmers are coached to swim their sets with a fixed amount of rest between each repeat, regardless of how fast, or slow, they swim each repeat. For example, a coach may give you a set of 10 x 50s on 15 seconds of rest. If it takes you 45 seconds to swim a 50, your true interval will be 1:00, 45 seconds of swimming and 15 seconds of rest. If you swim faster, let's say 35 seconds, then your true interval will be 0:50. Most of the time you will keep all the repeats around the same time, but you may decide to swim slower one day, perhaps your 50's take 1:00 to complete. On that day, your true interval is 1:15. This amount of variability and lack of control is problematic because it makes for inconsistent performances, and your coach doesn't really know how much work you're doing at each intensity.

What we want is to determine your intervals as quickly as possible. To do this, many coaches use what are called **test sets**. The classic test set is a "3000 for time." Exactly as it sounds, you swim 3000 yards (or meters) as fast as you can, trying to keep a steady pace throughout.

As a sprinter, I hated doing 3000's for time. They were incredibly boring. I always lost count, and I could never gauge my effort correctly, usually saving too much energy for the end. That means that I could have swum faster, meaning that my assigned intervals were too slow. So, when I became a coach, I looked for a simpler way to determine intervals for my swimmers.

Research scientist that I was, I started collecting data. After a lot of trial and error I devised a method of determining paces in three zones, Recovery Pace (RPE of 2-3), Base Pace (RPE 4-6), and LT Pace (RPE 7-8). All it requires is for you to swim a single, 100 (yards or meters) all-out sprint, from a push start.

I've collected data on numerous swimmers over the years, most recently with the help of three master's swimming programs in San Antonio, Dallas, and Portland, Oregon. Regardless of age, gender, or swimming experience, this method consistently works to set tight intervals for sets of 50's, 100's, and 200's. With the equations generated from this method, I have produced the reference tables in the back of the book.

To determine your paces for each of the three zones, find your time for your 100 sprint to the nearest second in the first column, and then find your pace ranges. For example, if your time for a 100 all out sprint is 1:13, your interval for a set of 10 x 100 at your recovery pace will be between 1:45-1:50. That means that you should be able to swim your repeat 100's in around 1:35-1:45, giving you 10-15 seconds of rest between each repeat. When you do a set of 10 x 100 at LT pace, your interval should be between 1:30-1:35. You should be able to swim these 100's in around 1:24-1:31, giving you 3-6 seconds of rest between each.

100 TIME	100 RECOVERY PACE (Borg 2–3, 10–15 sec rest)		
	Faster	Slower	Exact
1:13	1:45	1:50	1:47
	100 BASE PACE (Borg 4–6, 5–10 sec rest)		
	Faster	Slower	Exact
1:13	1:35	1:40	1:37
	100 LT PACE (Borg 7–8, 3–6 sec rest)		
	Faster	Slower	Exact
1:13	1:30	1:35	1:34

Most pools are equipped with pace clocks on either side of the pool. If you are using a pace clock, it is easiest to set your paces in 5 seconds increments. That's why I have provided a faster and slower pace. The better option is to use the exact time in the third column of each zone. This reflects the exact time that the equation generates for someone who swam a 1:13 for a 100 all out. Using your smart watch, program that time into your countdown timer.

Keep in mind that these pace ranges were produced with prediction equations that always have some error built into them. If you feel that your RPE is lower than 7-8 during your set of 10 x 100 at 1:30-1:35, try doing them at 1:25. This gives you a starting point. The next thing to remember is that you will get faster, and sometimes slower, over the course of a season. So, you need to do this test every 2–3 months. We will do it twice in the training programs to follow during weeks 3 and 8.

Using your heart rate, paces, and perceived exertion to structure your workouts will help you move from being an unfit person to a fit swimmer much faster than if you just hop in the pool and do a random number of laps. This method also provides a clear set of measurable goals that you can use to gauge your progress.

CHAPTER 11

Swimming Equipment:
THE INS AND OUTS

When it comes to buying swimming equipment, like any other product or service, you get what you pay for—at least, up to a point.

When I started competing in the triathlon in 2003, I was a poor doctoral student living off student loans and a very small salary as a teaching/research assistant. Just paying for entry fees was a challenge sometimes, so I had to be prudent with my equipment purchases. When it came to my bike, I spent around $900 on a road bike that I converted into a triathlon bike. I could've afforded a slightly pricier ride, but there wasn't going be enough benefit in terms of performance to justify the expense.

After joining my local triathlon club, I started attending group-training sessions. There was a clear division in the group in terms of bikes; those who had enough expendable income to afford bikes that were $4000 or more, and those like me, who could not.

In particular, there was this one guy. His name was Fred (we'll keep this story on a first name basis), and he rode a Cervello P5 that cost over $10,000. I have never been a brand name dropper, so I had no idea what any of us were riding. But Fred made sure to tell anyone who would listen about every piece of equipment he had *ever* purchased—how much time it would save him per mile, and of course, how much it cost. He wore the most expensive clothing, shoes, and sunglasses, and ate and drank only the latest supplements on the market.

The only problem was that Fred was as slow as molasses. During our 60–100-mile training rides, Fred would stick with us, babbling away about his latest purchases . . . at least, for the first ten miles while the rest of us warmed up. But as soon as the real riding started, the pace-line would form, the speed would get into the mid to upper 20s, and Fred would only make it through two or three turns pulling at the front of the pace-line, shielding the rest of us from the wind, before dropping out the back. This became a running joke and the proverb of "Don't be a Fred," was born. So, when it comes to buying your equipment for swimming, be reasonable. Don't buy the cheapest equipment just because it's inexpensive. Do your research and buy what works best for you and your budget. But, above all else, don't be a Fred.

GOGGLES

Next to your swimsuit, your goggles are the one piece of equipment that you will need for each practice session. The most important characteristic of goggles is that they be **watertight**. There is nothing more annoying that dealing with a slow leak while you're trying to concentrate on your stroke technique. So, avoid goggles that use any kind of foam between the plastic cup and your skin. The foam wears out quickly and begins to leak. You want goggles with a rubber seal or ones that have the plastic cup sitting directly on the skin around the eye.

The next characteristic is **comfort**. Your goggles may look really cool, but if they hurt when you wear them, they're useless. If you buy your gear at a brick-and-mortar store, ask to try on a pair of goggles. Make sure that you can adjust the centerpiece that goes over the bridge of the nose so that the cups are not too far apart or pinching on your nose.

The last thing to consider is **tinting**. If you are swimming inside, you will want clear lenses; if you are swimming outside, you will likely want some tinting on those lenses so that you don't have to squint if the sun is in your face. This can be a matter of personal preference, but is definitely a point to consider when making your purchase.

Now, I have no financial interest in any swim equipment companies, so any specific endorsements that I make are strictly from my opinions based on years of experience. My favorite type of goggles is what is called "Swedish." On the market since the early 1970s, they retail for around $5 for their basic pairs, and $15 if you want the flashy, metallic, tinted lenses. The goggles come unassembled; you get two cups, a short length of string to tie the cups together at the nose, a short rubber tube through which the string runs, and a long rubber strap that goes around your head, holding the cups in place. You can customize the fit until its perfect for you. It takes no more than 15 minutes.

My preferences aside, there are lots of great, affordable goggles on the market from Nike, TYR, Speedo, FINIS, and Sporti, just to name a few. A warning: don't get caught up in the anti-fog marketing nonsense. In my experience, the anti-fog technology is ineffective at best. Your goggles are going to get foggy as they get older and as the protective coating wears off. If your goggles are so foggy that you can't see the pace clock or the other end of the pool, it's time for some new goggles. You should not have to spend any more than $25 for a solid pair of goggles, and I urge you to look in the clearance rack. This is true for all pieces of equipment, but particularly goggles and suits.

SWIMSUITS

When buying a suit to practice in, head straight to the clearance rack, find a size that fits, walk to the checkout counter, buy it, and then go home.

It's really that simple. If you're more fashion conscious than am I, buy what you like, but don't get sold on how "fast" the suit is or is not. If you're going to wear it while swimming back and forth in a pool, the suit's drag coefficient doesn't matter. You can buy a good quality suit for less than $40. I would never spend more than $30 on a practice suit for me, or $60 on a suit for my daughter.

Now, if you are interested in racing, then buying a faster suit may be a good investment, up to a point. A regular practice suit will be made from nylon and 10–20% Lycra or Spandex to give it its elastic properties. These suits generate drag and soak up water like sponges, making you less buoyant. By contrast, "tech-suits" are engineered to reduce drag and water absorption, but you'll pay for that extra speed. Tech-suits range in cost from $200–$600.

FINS

All swimmers need a set of fins. I ask all my athletes to always have their own pair, and we use them for most, if not all practice sessions. When learning new techniques, the fins allow you to generate extra propulsive force with the legs, while the arms are moving more slowly through a new range of motion. Fins are fairly uniform in terms of their design, quality, and price. Some people like short fins, others like longer ones, like what you would use during scuba diving. I like fins that are in between those two extremes. A medium length fin extends three to eight inches beyond the toes, the longer the better. When you're trying on fins, go with ones that are little bigger if the next size down is too tight. This will reduce discomfort while kicking during long sets. A looser fin can cause blisters, but that's an easy fix: just keep an extra pair of ankle-high socks in your bag. You can get a good pair of fins for $25 or less.

One more note on fins. Although not a necessity, a few companies make monofins, where the feet are fused together into one big fin. This is a cool thing to use to improve your dolphin kick and butterfly stroke, but this should be considered a luxury purchase only. You can get one of these for $150-$200.

PULL BUOYS (Buoys)

Buoys are used to make your legs more buoyant, thus the name. It is a piece of foam shaped like an hourglass that you clench between your thighs while swimming with the arms only. The purpose is to keep the legs still while focusing on the arm pull of the stroke. This is not a piece of equipment that I use often. I typically use a buoy with new swimmers who have a hard time keeping their legs in line with the central axes of the body. I sometimes use a buoy when working on the breaststroke pull with a dolphin kick drill. I also use them with athletes who are nursing leg injuries, immobilizing the legs and letting them float instead of being dead weight. This is a $10 purchase.

PADDLES

Paddles are like fins for the hands and many coaches use them together with a buoy. Just like the fins strengthen the legs during kicking, paddles will strengthen the arms during a pull-only set. After fins, paddles are my favorite piece of equipment, but I say this as a *big* warning: Make sure that you use paddles that are the appropriate size *and* that you have had someone look at your stroke mechanics before you use them. Using paddles that are too big for you, or when you have terrible mechanics, can be a fast road to injury.

When making your selection, use the size chart and don't get distracted by the Fred in lane four swimming with the size 8 paddles when he should really be using size 3. Use the right size! This isn't a macho contest. Paddles range in price from $10-$30. TYR Catalysts are my brand and model of choice, but there are lots of different options on the market. Try these on in the shop or buy them from an online store that allows for returns if you don't like the fit. Once you've been cleared to use paddles, use them sparingly at first, building up to longer sets. No more than 20 percent of any workout done in the first month of swimming should be done while using paddles.

KICK BOARDS

This is another indispensable piece of equipment. Kick boards are akin to pull buoys, but they allow you to focus on your kick while keeping the upper body comfortably out of the water. If you are a new swimmer, you should be spending 20–30% of your time in the pool, kicking with a board. A quality kickboard shouldn't cost any more than $20.

SNORKELS

This is another piece of optional equipment, albeit one that is quite useful when trying to work on your freestyle technique. Instead of having to turn your head to breathe while swimming, you strap on the snorkel and focus on your stroke mechanics. Unlike the snorkels you used to get in a set with some cheap flippers and a scuba mask at your local toy store as a kid, these snorkels rise above the water, directly in front of your head, instead of off to one side. If you get one, be patient with yourself when using it the first time. It defies our natural instincts to inhale while our face is in the water. You may hyperventilate a little the first few times. If you get water in your snorkel, don't panic; just blast it out with one big exhalation. These range in price from $25-$45.

HIP ROTATOR

These are wonderful for swimmers of all levels. When swimming freestyle, you're moving around your central, longitudinal axis, during which you're rotating your whole body, not just your shoulders, around that axis with each stroke. The Hip Rotator is a belt that goes around the waist. A closed plastic tube with a plastic ball inside is attached to the back of the belt. As you roll from one side to the other, the ball rolls side to side as well, making an audible "click" each time it hits the wall of the tube. If you don't hear the click, you're not rolling enough. These retail for $50. A bit pricey, but worth it—this is *not* a Fred purchase.

DRAG SUITS

As your stroke becomes more efficient, you will burn fewer calories when swimming the same distance. This is great if you are looking to swim faster, but if you're mostly interested in weight loss, becoming more efficient can be a problem. Let's say that you swim a 3000-yard workout in June and again in December. You won't burn as many calories in December as you did in June. You can add more swimming to the workout, but if your time is limited there is another solution to this problem, make yourself less efficient by adding drag.

Drag suits are made from a heavier material than a normal swimsuit, and they have open pockets, two in the front and two in the back, that catch the water as you swim, slowing you down. You should only buy these if you have mastered your stroke and you want to burn more calories and increase strength. Because you wear a drag suit *over* your regular suit, both men and women wear the same design: briefs. These retail for around $40.

SMART WATCHES

A smart watch is a great piece of equipment to have for any sport. Some of the basic functions that you want are a count-down timer, and heart rate monitor. Watches that can monitor your heart rate variability and running or cycling distance are even better. When we get to the section on swimming intensity, you will need a count-down timer that you can set to any duration and is loud enough for you to hear it when it when you're in the pool. You also need it to have a heart rate monitor function that will chime when your heart rate goes over or falls under the ranges that you set for any given workout. Watches with these functions range in price from $200–$500.

Buying the appropriate equipment is a critical component of starting any new lifestyle change. It's important to be aware of cost, fit, utility, and aesthetics. Remember, the clearance rack is your best friend when getting started. Spend more on the critical items like goggles if you need to. Save your money on the more universal items like buoys, kickboards, and paddles. Express yourself with the fun stuff like a tie-dyed paisley swimsuit!

CHAPTER 12

Swimming Technique 101

F irst, a caveat: you can't learn how to participate in any sport by reading a book. The purpose of this chapter is to give you a brief history and technical description of each of the four competitive strokes, and to give you some basic pointers on some swimming drills you can do to improve your technique. In order to learn to swim safely and properly, you should find an experienced, certified swim coach. There are a few certifying organizations, but the two most prominent are the American Swimming Coaches Association (ASCA), and U.S. Masters Swimming. ASCA has five levels of certification, while U.S. Masters has four.

At a minimum, you want to find a coach who has achieved the criteria to be a level 1 certified coach in either organization. A simple way to find a coach or swim instructor is to use the "Club Finder" tab on the U.S. Masters Swimming website. If you're ready to jump right into a practice, most teams will let you try a week of practice for a nominal fee that is required to cover their insurance costs in case you get injured. If you need swim lessons, many coaches do that on the side, or at least know an instructor whom they can recommend. I find the best approach is to pick up the phone and call the person. Actually speaking to another person tends to be faster, and more productive than going back and forth over email or text.

A WORD ON STROKE DRILLS

All four strokes are complex, multi-joint movements that require you to learn several new motor pathways, training your brain to move your muscles the way you want them to. Add in the fact that you are doing this in a new environment, and it turns swimming into one of the toughest sports to master. Swimming drills are modifications of the normal stroke that allow you to break down the full stroke into single elements, arm drills, kick drills, breathing drills, etc. Once mastered, we can piece them all together to produce a better overall stroke. There are two mistakes that I see coaches and athletes make when it comes to drills:

- They do them only at the beginning of the season for two weeks and then not again until the following season.

- They race through them as fast as they can at the beginning of practice so they can get on with the "real" swimming.

Stroke drills are critically important to improving your stroke technique. If you're going to do them, do them right.

FREESTYLE (Front Crawl)

Although we most commonly use the term freestyle to describe the basic arm over arm stroke, the actual name of the stroke is the front crawl. Technically, the international governing body of swimming, Fédération Internationale De Natation (FINA), allows you to swim any of the four competitive strokes in a "freestyle" event. During my junior year of college, I had already qualified for our national championship meet in the 50-yard, 100-yard, and 200-yard freestyle events. You can only swim a maximum of three individual events, but my coach wanted to have as many options as possible for our team to score maximal points. So, during our conference championships, which were our last opportunity to swim official qualifying times, he had me swim a 200-yards Individual Medley (50-yards of butterfly, backstroke, breaststroke, and front crawl, in that order) during the 200-yard freestyle event, perfectly legal. I swam under the qualifying time by three seconds, but to my great relief, he didn't have me swim that event at nationals.

The two names are effectively synonymous, and you rarely hear anyone refer to freestyle as front crawl anymore. For simplicity, I will use the term freestyle from here out.

Arm Stroke

In the arm stroke, the arms should be in opposition, meaning that while one arm is out in front of the shoulders and head, the other has completed the underwater arm pull, and is at the level of the hips. Similarly, while one arm is pulling underneath the body, propelling water backward and moving the swimmer forward, the opposite arm is recovering through the air, leaving the water by the hips and travelling in an arc, entering the water near the head, and extending forward in front of the body.

Ideally, there is a delay of the stroke at the front, in other words the hands almost touch when your arms are extended in front of you. This allows for you to glide while taking a longer breath. As swimming speed increases, the delay gets shorter and shorter, because the stroke turnover increases. But, when looking at the fastest freestyle sprinters at the international level, the best ones still maintain a short glide. When an arm enters the water, it should extend directly in front of the shoulder before starting its pull. Imagine that you have a rod going straight through the midline of your body, starting at the base of your spine, and coming out the top of your head; your arms should never cross over that midline. Doing so makes your legs fish-tail behind as you as swim, causing excessive drag and pulling the legs out of position, limiting their effectiveness when kicking.

There are two commonly used methods when it comes to pulling the arms under the body. Some people keep their elbow straight, using the arm almost like an oar, moving water straight back. Others have a more fluid movement in the elbow, allowing the arm to move in a gentle S-shape, sweeping out, away from the head and then in toward the body, sweeping underneath the belly before moving back out again, exiting the water just past the hips. The purpose of the motion is to move as much water as possible, increasing the range of motion of the stroke. There is an obvious give and take here: if the S-shape motion is too slow, the stroke rate decreases, slowing the motion of the body through the water. Although the straight-arm method doesn't generate as much propulsive force as the S-shape method, the arms move faster through the water. It's a simple balancing act between range of motion and arm speed. The fastest, most efficient swimmers have enough arm strength and endurance to have the perfect combination of elbow flexibility (S-shaped movement) and arm speed.

Similarly, during the recovery phase while the arms are out of the water, there are two basic methods. The simplest recovery technique is to keep the arms almost fully extended with the elbows straight. Janet Evans was famous for using this technique during her dominant career as a distance swimmer in the late 80s and 90s. The other technique is to bend the elbow immediately after the hand exits the water at the hips, allowing the hand to swing forward like a pendulum, extending the elbow as the hand passes underneath, then reaching with the shoulder, placing the hand in the water near the head. Both techniques finish with the hand extending forward in front of the shoulder, allowing maximal glide and range of motion.

Breathing

Before going over breathing technique, let's cover the proper position of the head when you're *not* breathing. Returning to the idea of a rod from the base of your spine through the top of your head, if your head only moves around this rod, this is considered a neutral position. If you were floating in the prone position in the water, your face would be looking at the bottom of the pool. While swimming freestyle, you want your head to be just a little above neutral. If you're wearing a swimming cap, the water line should be at the level of the bottom of the cap on your forehead. If you hold your head any higher, you increase drag, any lower and you sink your shoulders.

As most people are righties, I'll describe how to breathe to the right side of the body first, but know that the process is exactly the same for the left side. The most common mistake new swimmers make is lifting their head out of the water with their face forward. This happens because they are afraid of getting water in their mouths, but it throws the body out of alignment, dropping the hips, making them sink. Again, you want to rotate around the central axis of your spine, turning your face to the right side, just enough to get about half of your mouth out of the water. As the fluid moves past your face, the surface tension of the water pulls the water line below your mouth, preventing much water from entering. Starting with your right hand in the extended position, press down on the water as you begin to pull your arm back, initiating the pull stroke. As you press on the water, this provides enough lift to get your head out of the water high enough for you to rotate your face to the right and take a breath. The rotation should come from the entire body and not just the head. Your face stays exposed from the time you start your arm pull to just before the end of the recovery phase.

Next is the part everyone hates, at least initially. While your face is in the water, you need to be slowly exhaling through your nose and mouth. This accomplishes two things:

1. You keep any water from entering your nose, which is a terrible feeling.

2. When it comes time to turn your face out of the water, you don't have to waste any time exhaling. Most new swimmers will hold their breath until the bitter end, making them both exhale and inhale in one go.

There are two camps when it comes to breathing frequency: those who believe that you must breathe to both sides (bilateral breathing), alternating every three to five strokes, and those who think that breathing to one side every two to four strokes is fine (unilateral breathing). Personally, I find unilateral breathing makes the most sense. There is no other sport during which you have to hold your breath and breathe to both sides of your body. I want to breathe as often as possible, especially when I'm in water! Although many will say that bilateral breathing reduces the risk of over-usage injuries of the shoulders, there is no published scientific evidence to support this idea.

Kicking

Freestyle is done with a flutter kick. Just like the arms, the legs move in opposition, while one leg is kicking down, the other is moving back up. The kick should be initiated at the hip. New swimmers tend to keep their hips tight and kick with only the lower half of the legs. If you think of the leg as a lever, the longer it is, the more water it can move. By kicking from the knee, you have chopped your lever in half, not to mention that you are not using the huge leg muscles of the quads and hamstrings.

The motion of the leg should look like a whip, with the wave of motion starting at the hip and rolling down the leg, past the knee, and cracking at the point of the toes breaking the surface of the water. This brings me to my final point on the freestyle stroke. Although the feet will break the surface, they should just barely do so. If you bend at the knee so much that your leg is exposed at mid-calf, when you kick down through the air, you are not generating any propulsive force. This is true for the kick of each of the respective strokes.

If you want a quick history lesson, look no further than David Berkoff. An American backstroker from the 1988 Seoul Summer Olympics, Berkoff was the world record holder at the time, having revolutionized the event by staying underwater for the first 35 meters (in a 50-meter pool) doing dolphins kicks while everyone else was on the surface swimming. While under the surface of the water, he could kick both down *and* up, doubling the propulsive force of his kick, while staying is a streamlined position. Soon everyone was using the technique, appropriately named the Berkoff Blastoff, and more than half of the race was competed underwater. Not exactly spectator friendly ... but undeniably effective. (In the early 1990s, FINA made a new rule that, regardless of the stroke, you could only stay underwater for 15 meters.)

The point being, if your arms or legs leave the water during the arm pull or kick, you lose propulsion. So, when you're practicing your kick, keep your feet under the water.

FREESTYLE STROKE DRILLS

Finger-Drag Freestyle

The underwater arm pull for this drill is the same as it is for the regular stroke. But, as the hand exits the water by the hips, bend your elbow, keeping the tips of your fingers in the water and drag them forward, underneath your elbow, extending your hand in front of your shoulder, before starting your arm pull again.

The purpose of this drill is to promote an arm recovery that sweeps parallel to the body's centerline. As we discussed earlier, arm recovery through the air can be achieved with either a straight-arm technique, or with the hand swinging underneath the bent elbow like a pendulum. In either case, we want the hand to sweep through air, in a line parallel to the centerline, and not in a horizontal arc, just above the surface of the water.

This accomplishes three things:

1. It keeps the hands away from the choppy surface of the water where they can hit little waves.

2. It promotes extension of the arms in straight lines in front of the shoulders and prevents them from crossing the centerline in front of the face.

3. It reduces strain on the shoulder that is common with a wide, sweeping stroke.

Catch-up Freestyle

The stroke technique, both during the arm pull and recovery is the same as during the regular stroke. But, in order to emphasize the delay at the front of the stroke, you will touch your hands together in front of your body between strokes. For example, your left hand has just finished its recovery and is fully extended in front of your shoulder. Before it begins its pull, allow the right hand to finish its pull and recovery, and touch your hands together before starting the arm pull of the left hand.

I like to have new swimmers do this drill while wearing a pair of fins, as they help maintain propulsion while emphasizing the glide between strokes. As you get stronger as a swimmer, you can take off the fins. The purpose of this drill is to slow down the stroke rate, emphasizing full extension of the arms. Many swimmers feel that they will sink if they don't maintain a constant, fast cadence. This is not an efficient way to swim. Every time we move our limbs away from the centerline, we increase the amount of drag imposed on the body. So, increasing the duration of the glide allows you to save energy. Now, there is an obvious breakpoint, if you don't pull, you stop moving. So, you have to balance the gliding time with the propulsion time. This drill helps you find that sweet spot.

Six-Kick Freestyle

Many new swimmers have a flat freestyle stroke. By this, I mean they position their bodies in the water like they are lying on a surfboard. The arm pulls look as though they are paddling; shallow, and wide. The recovery phase is parallel to the water's surface; the arms swing wide and enter the water well outside the line of the shoulder. All the propulsive force comes from the shoulders, with no help from the core (abdominal and back muscles). Ideally, we want the shoulders, and the rest of the body, to roll gently, side-to-side. For example, as your left arm begins its pull under the body, your body rolls onto your left side at an angle of 35–45° relative to the surface of the water. The left shoulder is completely submerged under the water, while the right shoulder rises above the water during its recovery phase. To move you from flat swimming to rolling side-side, I teach the six-kick freestyle drill to exaggerate the movement of the body.

Again, for new swimmers, this drill is best done with fins. Push off from the wall with your arms extended in front of your shoulders and your hands together. The arms should be squeezing your head, which should be in a neutral position, with your imaginary rod traveling through the spine and out the top of the head. This is a basic streamline position. Take one arm pull with your right arm and then roll onto your left side to 90°, keeping your left arm extended in front of your shoulder, and your right hand resting on your right hip. Now that you are on your left side, all the propulsive force in coming from your kick. After six, slow flutter kicks on your left side, start your left arm pull and roll to your right side. At the same time, your right arm completes its recovery phase. This is when you take your breath as well. Stay on your right side and count out six kicks again. You can breathe every stroke while doing this drill.

The purpose of this drill is to emphasize that the body should roll from side to side around the central, longitudinal axis.

This accomplishes three things:

1. The rolling motion engages the core muscles, generating significantly more force than can be generated by the arms alone.

2. The range of motion of the stroke is significantly increased, meaning that you can move more water and generate more propulsion.

3. You rotate your head into a position above the water line that allows you to take a longer breath.

BACKSTROKE

The backstroke was first used in competition in the 1900 Paris Olympic games. It is the favorite stroke of many people because their face is out of the water the entire time and they can breathe whenever they like. The basic elements of the stroke are effectively an inverted version of freestyle. Similar to freestyle, I want you to imagine that you have a rod running through your spine, this time, exiting at the base of your neck, with your head resting on it at a very gentle angle. Placing your head too far back drops the shoulders and washes water over your face. Lifting your head too high makes the hips drop, creating drag and slowing you down.

Arm Stroke

The backstroke must be done with a straight-arm recovery, with the hand exiting the water next to the hip, with the thumb up and palm facing inward toward the body. The arm travels in an arc parallel to the centerline. As the hand moves through the air, it rotates so that the pinky enters the water first, and the palm is facing away from the body. Just remember, thumb out, pinky in. Like freestyle, backstroke is not to be swum flat on your back. You need to rotate the body around your central axis to 35–45°, keeping the head perfectly still. Don't let it rock from side to side or bounce up and down.

The arm pull of backstroke requires an S-shaped sweep of the hand, with the elbow slightly bent. After the right hand enters the water, pinky-first, palm-out, and the shoulder completely submerged, the elbow bends, bringing the arm closer to the body. From this position, the hand sweeps up toward the surface of the water and then pushes down toward the legs, exiting next to the hips with the thumb up. If you try this without the shoulder roll, flat on your back, as the hands sweeps over the top of its arc, the fingers will break the surface of the water. This is a tell-tale sign of poor shoulder rotation, and since your hand is now pushing air, and not water, you lose propulsion.

Breathing

Since your face is out of the water, technically you can breathe whenever you want to, but it is best to breathe in rhythm with your stroke cadence. I typically breathe in while my right arm is in the recovery phase, and out when my left arm is recovering.

Kicking

The backstroke's kick is the mirror image of the freestyle kick. It initiates at the hip and whips through the knee, finishing at the toes. Having your head slightly elevated allows the legs to sink ever so slightly, keeping the feet under surface of the water. Another reason to not lay the head too far back is that this results in your feet breaking the surface of the water. Remember, moving water generates propulsion. Moving air does nothing.

BACKSTROKE DRILLS

Six-Kick Backstroke

The purpose of this drill is the same as it is for freestyle: we want to increase the range of motion in the body roll. Since backstroke kick tends to be weaker than freestyle kick, I always have my new swimmers use fins during this drill. The fins provide enough propulsion to keep you moving so you don't feel like you're going to sink, and they add enough resistance to keep the knee from bending too much.

Push off from the wall on your back in a streamlined position. Let the left hand move down to the left hip as you roll onto your right side at a 90° angle. Your head should still be looking straight up at the ceiling, in line with your central axis. Kick six, long, slow kicks, and then start your right arm pull, taking the hand deep before bending the elbow, and sweeping the hand in an arc that starts up towards the surface of the water, goes over the elbow, and then pushes down toward the toes. At the same time, the left hand leaves the water by the hip, thumb-first. As the left arm recovers in a large arcing motion, it remains straight. The hand rotates and enters the water pinky-first as you roll to your left side. You finish with your head in the same position, looking straight up at the ceiling of the pool (or sky). Maintain your kick throughout the drill.

Two-Arm Backstroke

The purpose of this drill is to emphasize the straight-arm recovery over the water, with the thumbs exiting the water by the hips and the pinkies entering, in line with the shoulders. Do this while wearing your fins. As you get stronger, you can do this drill without them. Because both arms will be moving together, synchronously, side-by-side, you will swim the drill flat on your back. That means that you must modify the arm pull, keeping the elbows straight, using the arms like oars.

Push off from the wall on your back in a streamlined position and start your kick. Keep the kick going the entire time so that you don't lose propulsion during the drill. Pull both hands down to the hips in sweeping arcs that are parallel to the surface of the water. As both hands exit the water, thumbs-up, keep your elbows locked and follow the path of the hands with your head as they pass over the shoulders, then extend in front of the head, entering the water pinky-first. Stay in this position for a count of four or five kicks before repeating.

BREASTSTROKE

Breaststroke is the oldest of the four strokes. When watching someone swim the stroke, it's somewhat reminiscent of watching a frog swim, or at least kick through the water. Being that the kick is the toughest part of the breaststroke to master, try to imagine what a frog kicking looks when you try the breaststroke kick for the first time.

For most, breaststroke is the easiest of the four strokes to swim. Its popularity is because a derivation of the stroke allows you to keep your head above water the entire time. The earliest published illustrations of breaststroke date to 1538, when Nicolaus Wynmann published the *Colymbetes*, a book about swimming safety, in his attempt to reduce the frequency of drownings that occurred prior to the Renaissance. Wynmann also described ways to make floatation devices from inflated cow stomachs and bladders. Yum! In more recent history, breaststroke was first competed in the 1904, St. Louis Olympics.

Arm Stroke

The arm pull begins in the streamline position. The hands move apart and press down on the water. At their widest, the arms are in a position that makes the body look like the letter "Y" when observed from above. Immediately after the arms are at their widest and deepest points, the elbows bend, sweeping the hands under the chest at a line parallel to the shoulders. The downward motion of the hands provides lift, allowing the head and shoulders to come above the surface of the water. This is when you take your breath. The combined downward and backward movements of the arms generate the propulsive force to move the body forward. During this phase, the legs are straight behind you. They do not do their part until just before you begin the recovery phase of the stroke. The hands come together, under the chest, when the shoulders and head are at their highest point during the breath. From there, the hands "shoot" forward rapidly and extend out in front of your body as your head comes down between your arms. It is the kick that allows you to maintain forward propulsion during the "shoot" phase of the arm stroke.

So, unlike freestyle and backstroke, during which the arms and legs are moving simultaneously, during both breaststroke and butterfly, there is a division of labor. The rhythm of the breaststroke is pull, kick, glide . . .

pull, kick, glide... The glide is done with the head in a neutral position and the arms extended, in order to reduce drag. The duration of the glide can be long for slower, longer distance swims, or extremely short during short-distance sprints.

Kicking

Again, think about a frog kicking. The kick starts with the legs fully extended, feet plantar-flexed so that the toes are pointing straight behind you. The recovery phase of the kick begins, when you bend the knees, drawing the heels to the butt, while the thighs move apart. The feet finish this phase in dorsiflexion (the ankles bent at 90°), and the heels close to the butt. The actual distance of the feet from the backside is variable between swimmers, but the closer they get (within reason) the more propulsive force they generate as they travel back to the starting position.

When the legs have reached the fully recovered position, they are ready to start the power phase of the kick. At this point the hands are together, under the chest, with the head and shoulders at their highest positions, immediately after the arm pull phase of the stroke, and right before the shoot. The power phase of the kick begins with the knees and feet flexed, and the legs spread apart. The motion of the kick, whips the feet around, and back, finishing with the knees and ankles fully extended, and the feet together, toes pointing to the back wall.

The timing of the three phases of the breaststroke is critical for a fast, efficient stroke. Don't be impatient and skip the glide. At the same time, don't glide so long that you start to slow down. Remember, pull, kick, glide!

BREASTSTROKE DRILLS

Two Kicks, One Pull

This drill is just like it sounds. After a pull, kick, glide, you add a second kick, then go back into your arm pull phase. During the second kick, you remain in a streamlined position, with your arms extended and your head in a neutral position. The purpose of the drill is to emphasize the glide phase of the stroke.

Breaststroke with a Flutter Kick

Again, self-explanatory. Take a normal breaststroke arm pull while your feet are doing the flutter kick quickly. This will eliminate your glide completely and the purpose of the drill is to emphasize the shoot phase of your recovery. The flutter kick allows you to shoot your hands out in front of you more rapidly than when doing breaststroke kick. Try doing it with fins the first few times. Remember, this is just a drill that we do to speed up the recovery phase of the arm stroke.

Breaststroke with a Dolphin Kick

Aptly named. Take a normal breaststroke arm pull and as you shoot your hands forward, do one big dolphin kick, then glide for a slightly longer distance than normal. The purpose of this drill is to allow you to get your shoulders and head out of the water a little higher before starting the shoot phase. The higher the shoulders, the faster they come down into the glide. Do this drill while wearing your fins.

BUTTERFLY

The butterfly is typically considered the most difficult stroke to master. Of the four strokes, the butterfly is the youngest. It was first competed in the 1956 Melbourne Olympics. Interestingly, the butterfly stroke was derived from breaststroke. Because the slowest phase of the breaststroke is the shoot, as the arms extend forward through the water, people started to throw their arms forward *over* the water. Over time, the shoot phase was eliminated completely, and the arms recovered over the water, rotating around the shoulder, just over the surface of the water, i.e. the modern butterfly arm stroke. But this version of breaststroke maintained the frog kick, and as the stroke evolved further, the frog kick was replaced with a dolphin kick. FINA accepted this final version of butterfly as a separate, unique stroke in 1952.

Like breaststroke, the fulcrum of the butterfly stroke rotates around an imaginary rod traveling through the body, from one side to the other, at the level of the hips. Unlike breaststroke, during which there is 1:1 ratio for the arm pull and kick, the butterfly has one arm pull, one big, propulsive kick, and a second, smaller kick, that allows the hips to rise and recover before the big kick. So, the rhythm for butterfly is pull, big kick, small kick.

Arm Stroke

The arm stroke for butterfly, although the toughest in terms of upper body strength, is ironically the least technical of the four strokes. The stroke starts as the hands enter the water simultaneously, either directly in line with the shoulders or just outside that line. The hands should enter the water, fingertips first, and with a slight pitch of the wrists, pointing the fingers down to the floor of the pool.

The catch phase of the arm pull starts by pressing the chest into the water. This brings the hips up, positioning them for the big kick. With the chest pressing down, the arms press down and out, generating lift, and bringing the head and shoulders above the water. As the hands sweep in a subtle S-shape movement under the body and back to the hips, this provides the forward propulsive force that moves the body forward and allows you to start to lift your head for the breath. The hands travel all the way back to the level of the hips at which point they exit water, palms up, to begin the recovery phase of the stroke.

During the recovery phase of the stroke, the hands sweep around from the hips to the entry position described at the start of the stroke. The arms should be fully extended throughout the recovery phase, and they should be as close as possible to the water, without skipping along the surface. This is the sticking point of the stroke for most people because the arms are no longer generating propulsive force and without timing the kick correctly, they come to a stop in the water. This is where the big kick comes in. As the arms sweep forward during the recovery phase, the legs do the big dolphin kick, providing the propulsive force and preventing the body from stalling.

Breathing

The head position for the breath is most often looking straight down the pool. The head begins to rise as the hands sweep underneath the body and should be completed, at its highest points, as the hands begin the recovery phase of the stroke, with the legs driving the body forward. Once the breath is completed, the head should start dropping. This begins when the arms are at 90 degrees to the central axis of the body, i.e., straight out to the sides. The head should enter the water face down, in a neutral position, at the same time as the hands enter the water in front of the body.

One common mistake is to raise the head too high, exposing the chest, and dropping the hips. This causes two problems:

1. It increases drag.

2. It changes the direction of propulsion from the horizontal plane to the vertical plane. You want to be moving forward, through the water. Moving up and down is bad.

Kicking

Butterfly utilizes a dolphin kick, during which the legs must move in the same direction at the same time. Although the feet do not have to be together, if they switch positions, that is considered a flutter kick, and is illegal. For example, you can do a dolphin kick with the right foot slightly above the left. As long as they stay in that orientation, all is well. But if you switch it so that the left foot is above the right, that one kick is a flutter kick, it is best to keep the feet parallel to each other in the same plane.

There are two kicks during the stroke cycle of butterfly. The big kick starts with the hips high in the water. The kick initiates at the hips and whips down the legs through the knees, to the toes. The hips drive down to start the wave of motion along the legs. The second, smaller kick is done to bring the hips back up, preparing them to start another big kick. The smaller kick happens a short time after the big kick, as the chest is pressing down on the water, and the hands are beginning their catch phase of the arm pull.

BUTTERFLY DRILLS

The simplest modification to the stroke that will help you learn to swim it more efficiently is to swim with fins. The extra push from the legs really reduces the strain on the arms and slows the timing down so that you can feel each part of the stroke. I would spend the first month of swimming butterfly wearing the fins, and once you feel strong enough, take the fins off and do one length of butterfly at a time, working on technique and timing.

One-Arm Butterfly

You can do this drill with or without fins, but again, for the first month, I suggest you use the fins. Push off the wall in the streamline position, doing three powerful dolphin kicks to bring you to the surface with reasonable forward momentum. While keeping the left arm extended in front of the shoulder, initiate the stroke sequence with the right arm only. You can breathe straight ahead (preferable), or turn your head to the side like you would do during freestyle. Swim the entire length with one arm, and then switch arms at the turn and swim back with the other arm.

The purpose of this drill is to allow you to maintain your body position with one arm extended, while focusing on perfecting the movement of your stroking arm. Follow the motion of your hand as it starts the catch phase, passes underneath the body, exits at the hip, and sweeps around during the recovery. Focus on the undulation of the upper body and head. The chest should drive down as the catch phase starts, bringing the hips up, readying them for the big kick, etc.

1-1-2 Drill

This drill is the next step in the progression of learning the full stroke. You take one stroke with the right arm as the left arm stays in its extended position. After completing the right arm stroke, take a stroke with the left arm, while the right arm stays extended. After completing the left arm stroke, take a stroke with both arms. The legs kick normally throughout the drill. Continue this pattern.

The purpose of this drill is to perfect the motion of each of the arms separately, *and* together, little by little, moving toward swimming the complete stroke with better technique.

Being able to legally swim all four of the competitive strokes is import-ant because it allows you to design more interesting workouts and reduces the likelihood of over usage injuries that commonly occur when you do the same activity day after day. Remember, the best path to learning to swim each stroke correctly is to find a coach who can get you started.

PART 3

PRACTICAL APPLICATIONS & NEXT STEPS

CHAPTER 13

Basic Nutrition for Swimming Performance

Nutrition and exercise go hand in hand, a topic which I have researched and written about extensively. (For a more in-depth explanation of these topics, I invite you to read my first book, *Exercise Ain't Enough: HIIT, Honey, and the Hadza.*) Here, I provide an overview of the basics of nutrition, as well as my recommended diet for weight loss, weight management, and general health—the Mediterranean diet.

MACRONUTRIENTS

Macronutrients are differentiated from micronutrients based on the quantities of each that we consume per day. The average person eats kilograms worth of macronutrients every day, but we rarely consume more than a few hundred milligrams of any micronutrient. Another distinguishing characteristic between the two is that we metabolize macronutrients to make ATP (the energy currency of all living things), while micronutrients play critical roles as coenzymes and cofactors in the different metabolic pathways. In other words, micronutrients help us breakdown macronutrients, extracting energy from them in the form of calories. But micronutrients are not themselves metabolized to make ATP.

Fat

Dietary fats are the most energy dense of the three macronutrients at 9 calories/gram. Because of this, fat is our preferred fuel source during rest and low-intensity exercise. When we use the word fat in reference to nutrition, what we are really talking about are large molecules called triglycerides. A triglyceride is made of a backbone of glycerol and three long-chain fatty acids. We store fat as triglycerides in fat cells (adipocytes), which are located under our skin (subcutaneous), in our muscles (intramuscular), and lining our abdominal organs (visceral). When we metabolize fats, it's only the fatty acids that are broken down to make ATP; most of the glycerol is recycled to make new triglycerides.

There are two basic structures of fatty acids: saturated and unsaturated. **Saturated fats** are mainly found in animal products, such as meat, eggs, dairy. **Unsaturated fats** come from plants including olives, avocados, nuts, seeds, and from fish. Butter is a good example of a saturated fat that is typically solid at room temperature. By contrast, unsaturated fat is liquid at room temperature. Some examples include olive, vegetable, and fish oil.

For decades, saturated fats were vilified as being unhealthy. They were stripped out of many prepared and packaged "fat free" foods and replaced by sugar. These products played a significant role in the obesity crisis that started in the 1980s and continues today. Both saturated and unsaturated fats are part of a healthy diet. They are digested and absorbed more slowly than carbohydrates, reducing cravings between meals. I suggest that fats comprise around 35–40% of your daily calories, with about 10% coming in the form of saturated fats, and the rest from unsaturated fats.

Carbohydrates (Carbs)

Dietary carbs are a class of macronutrient ranging in size from the very small, simple sugars (glucose, fructose, and galactose), all the way up to huge polymers of thousands of glucose molecules called starches. We can store glucose in the liver and muscles, in the form a different polymer called glycogen. Carbs provide four calories/gram, but they burn much faster than do fats, so we tend to use carbs preferentially during high-intensity exercise when our need for rapid ATP production is highest.

As happened with fats in the 1980s and 1990s, there has recently been a push to make all food "low-carb" or even "no-carb." Unfortunately, this has been just as misguided as the fat-free craze that preceded it. Eliminating all carbs means removing healthy foods from your diet that have lots of starch and fiber, like fruits, vegetables, and grains. The fact of the matter is that we would not do very well without carbs in our diet. Our brain requires a minimum amount of glucose to always be on hand and will direct the body to turn protein into glucose if blood sugar levels fall too low.

A better goal is to try and reduce, but not eliminate, the amount of sugar in your diet. There is clear evidence that over-consumption of sugar leads to weight gain. The excess sugar that we take in is simply converted to fat and stored. The best practice is to eat several servings or raw, whole foods including fruits, vegetables, and whole grains. I suggest that carbo-hydrates comprise around 45% of your daily calories, with only 5% coming from simple sugars, and the rest coming from more complex carbs like starches. Although starches will eventually be broken down to simple sugars, that takes time, and the delay in digestion of larger, complex carbs allows us to feel satiated.

Protein

Like carbs, proteins generate four calories/gram when metabolized. Like fats, proteins are digested and absorbed more slowly than carbs, making us feel full for a longer time. The basic building blocks of proteins are called amino acids, of which there are twenty. Our bodies can synthesize 11 of these 20 amino acids, making them non-essential; however, the other nine are considered essential and we must consume them in our diet. Sources of protein that contain all nine essential amino acids are considered "complete" proteins. The best examples are animal proteins, eggs, fish, dairy products, and plant foods like quinoa and soy.

Our bodies don't store protein; all our proteins are functional. Because of this, under normal circumstances we metabolize negligible amounts of protein to make ATP. However, if glucose levels are too low for a few days, perhaps during a fast, or after starting a new diet, the liver starts to make glucose from protein. So, it is important to make sure that your meals and snacks contain adequate amounts of complete proteins. I suggest that proteins comprise around 15–20% of your daily calories. You can safely consume 2 grams/kg of body weight. For an average male weighing 70 kg (154 pounds), this equates to 1/3 of a pound of protein per day.

MICRONUTRIENTS

Vitamins

Vitamins are either water-soluble (C, and the B complex vitamins) or fat-soluble (A, E, D, and K). We can store the fat-soluble vitamins in our adipocytes and liver. Because of this, they can be toxic if we consume too much of them. By contrast, we do not store water-soluble vitamins. That's why your urine looks somewhat neon yellow when you take a multivitamin.

- Vitamin C acts as an antioxidant, protecting the cells from free radicals, damaging chemicals that are made during metabolism. It is also active in the production of collagen, the most abundant protein in the body, which is found in our skin, bones, and gums. Vitamin C deficiency results in thin skin that bruises easily, and loose teeth, a condition called Scurvy.

- Vitamin B has a variety of forms, with eight B complex vitamins. They play vital roles in helping us metabolize macronutrients into ATP, and maintaining bodily functions including cell growth, digestion, brain function, muscle tone, and cardiovascular health.

- Vitamin A is used to make the pigment that captures light in the retina of the eye. Deficiency can lead to night blindness.

- Vitamin E is used by the body as another potent antioxidant.

- Vitamin D stimulates the intestines to absorb calcium. This is why we fortify milk with Vitamin D; it increases the amount of calcium that we can move from the milk to our bones.

- Vitamin K is necessary for the clotting process after we sustain an injury or bleed.

Minerals

Minerals have numerous varied roles in the body. A good example of this is calcium. The "cement" part of our bones is called hydroxyapatite, a mineral compound made from calcium and phosphorous. We also need calcium in order to trigger our muscles to contract, and to allow for impulses to travel from one neuron to another. Other examples of important minerals are iron, iodine, sodium, and potassium.

- Iron is part of both hemoglobin and myoglobin, pigments that bind to O_2, moving it through the blood and into muscles, respectively.

- Iodine is part of our thyroid hormones that stimulate our metabolism.

- Sodium and potassium are required for the conduction of nerve impulses and the contraction of our muscles.

Phytochemicals

Phytochemicals are most easily identified in fruits and vegetables with vibrant colors, orange, red, purple. Phytochemicals are plant-derived nutrients that act as potent anti-inflammatories, antioxidants, and pain relievers.

Fiber

Finally, there is dietary fiber. Since we cannot digest fiber, it is not really considered food or a nutrient, but it still plays an extremely important, and undervalued role in our health. There are two types of fiber, soluble and insoluble. Humans cannot digest either form, but both provide important health benefits.

When soluble fiber is mixed with water in the stomach and small intestine it takes on the texture and weight of jelly. This slows the movement of food through these two organs, making us feel full, longer. Soluble fiber also binds to cholesterol in the small intestine, carrying it out in feces, lowering our circulating cholesterol levels. Finally, soluble fiber serves as a food source for the good bacteria living in our large intestine. When these good bacteria eat soluble fiber, they produce a substance called Butyrate, which is then metabolized by the cells lining our gut, keeping the barrier between our intestines and the inside of our body strong and reducing inflammation. Soluble fiber is found in beans, fruits, and oats.

Then, there is insoluble fiber. This is what we call "roughage." In plants, insoluble fibers are structural; think of plant stalks and the bran of grains. Insoluble fibers are completely indigestible, so they move right through our digestive system like a broom, sweeping out all the leftover waste. This speeds the transit time through the large intestine, keeping us "regular," and potentially reducing the risk of colon cancer. Foods rich in insoluble fiber include the skins of fruits and vegetables, root vegetables, green leafy vegetables, and whole grains.

Unfortunately, the American diet is woefully inadequate when it comes to fiber intake. Although we should be taking in around 30-35 grams/day, with no upper limit, Americans, on average, only take in about 15 grams/day. This is an easy fix that can have a major, positive impact on your health.

POST-WORKOUT SNACKS

Regardless of what kind of exercise you do, be it land-based or swimming, aerobic or resistance training, it is always a good idea to have a post-workout snack within 30 minutes of finishing.

There are three reasons for this:

1. The carbs in the snack will restore your glycogen stores in your liver and muscles.
2. The amino acids in the snack will stimulate protein synthesis in the muscles.
3. The snack will reduce your hunger so that you are less likely to overeat during your next meal.

The composition of the snack is important. It needs to contain all three macronutrients, in particular protein and carbs. Research has clearly shown that when protein and carbs are consumed together in a post-workout snack, muscles absorb both nutrients more rapidly than when they are consumed separately. The fat in the snack is there for flavor and to slow absorption in the small intestine, making you feel full, longer, reducing your hunger pangs.

The perfect snack should have about 20-25 grams of protein, 6-10 grams of carbs (only 1-2 grams from sugar), and about 7-10 grams of fat (mostly unsaturated). If we max out all these numbers, i.e., 25 grams of protein, 10 grams of carbs, and 10 grams of fats, we get 210 calories, a reasonable amount for a post-workout snack. Be sure to account for these calories when you're planning your daily intake. They aren't free, or extra calories.

Finally, pick a snack that tastes good and has a texture that your stomach can handle after a swimming workout. For example, I like to drink a shake. You can buy a huge tub of whey protein powder and put a few scoops into a shaker cup—just add water and you're done. And when you find one or two snacks that you really like, order them in bulk online and save some money!

Food should be nourishing and sustaining. It provides the raw materials needed to grow, repair, and rejuvenate the mind, body, and soul. But to be sure, food is more than just fuel, it should be savored, craved, and enjoyed. If you take just a little time, you can find foods that will do all of these things at the same time. Use these simple pointers to help you establish a new relationship with food as you begin this new journey of swimming for life.

CHAPTER 14

Strength Training for Swimmers

Y ou cannot teach someone strength training exercises in a book. Our objective for this section is not to train you in proper strength training, but rather to educate you on what parts of the body to focus on and explain why these exercises are important. That way, when you do meet with a coach or start a strength training program, you'll understand each exercise and the impact it has on your body.

On that note, any motion that is repeated—like drills—has the potential to cause injury. This occurs as a result of two factors:

1. The muscles that are repeatedly contracted become chronically fatigued and more susceptible to injury.

2. The muscles on the other side of the joint become comparably weaker, causing an imbalance in the joint, making it more susceptible to injury.

The best example of this is with long distance runners. Running is an exercise driven by the quads. Because of this, many runners have chronically weak hamstrings. The imbalance of strength between the two muscle groups can pull the knees and hips out of alignment, causing injury to the muscles and joints. The solution is to have runners do some basic strengthening exercises of the hamstrings and the peripheral stabilizer muscles of the legs and lower back.

By contrast, swimming is an exercise driven by the arms, shoulders, and upper back, specifically, the triceps, pectorals, deltoids, and lats (the big muscles of the upper back that contract when using the lat pull down machine). You may notice that younger swimmers have poor posture, slouching forward. It looks like their chest muscles are so tight that they pull the shoulders forward. This imbalance frequently leads to over usage injuries of the front of the shoulder, and to a lesser extent, the elbows. I strongly recommend that my swimmers do a series of exercises that strengthen the muscles surrounding the shoulder, upper back, and the core. Since the anterior muscles are already stronger than the posterior muscles, I use a 1:2 ratio (anterior to posterior) of the reps that are done with each muscle group respectively.

I recommend doing these exercises before your workout, as part of your warm-up, or on a non-swimming day. I like to do three sets of 6–20 repetitions. Start with 6 repetitions of each and add 2 additional reps to each set per week, until you get to 20 reps per set. It's ok to pick a routine that you like and keep doing it for several weeks. But, if you get bored after two weeks, change the exercises.

Some exercises that I recommend for swimmers looking to build strength include:

Bicep Curls	External Rotation
Triceps Extensions	Fire Hydrants
Squatting Arm Rows	Side-Step Squats
Chest Press	One-Leg Donkey Kicks
One Arm L-Pull	Sit-ups
Butterfly Pulls	One-Leg V-ups
Freestyle Pulls	Twisting Heel-Touches
Internal Rotation	Supermans

BASIC DRYLAND EQUIPMENT FOR SWIMMING RESISTANCE TRAINING

There are numerous implements that you can use for dryland training, but for our purposes here, we are going to keep things really simple.

To get started you need four pieces of equipment:

- **A pair of resistance bands.** These are linked together at the far end with a nylon strap that you can anchor to a post or table leg. The other end has two plastic handles to grip. There are several brands to choose from, but just for reference, my favorite is StrecthCordz. Remember, start with a lighter resistance, and move up later. These run about $50.

- **A mini-band or resistance loop**. These are shorter and thicker than your usual resistance bands. They are meant to go around the knees or ankles. You can get a good one for about $15–$20.

- **Yoga mat**. This is optional, but a nice thing to have. You can get one for $10-$20.

- **Medicine ball**. Start with a 5 or 10-pound ball and get heavier ones if you need them. While optional, I use these with core exercises all the time to great effect.

Strength training is a critical component of any fitness routine. Resistance training is both a supplement that will improve your swimming performance and the best way to reduce the likelihood of injuries. Find what works best for you and stick with it.

CHAPTER 15

Cross Training and Open Water Swimming

AVOIDING PLATEAUS AND BURNOUT

Having been a competitive swimmer and coach for many years, I have seen a lot of young kids—who were considered the next big thing when they were 11—get left behind by their peers when they turn 14. In some instances, these kids had an early growth spurt that was not followed by another of the same magnitude, but more often than not, what I see are kids who get burned out on swimming.

Burnout is both psychological and physiological and it can happen to anyone, at any stage of life, in any sport. The best cure for burnout is to mix things up. Over the last 30 years, parents have decided to specialize their children in one sport instead of changing sports with the seasons. The same can be said for adults, too. Obviously, I am an advocate for the sport of swimming. However, I am also an advocate for balance. That means that on your non-swimming days, you should try mixing in some cycling, running, or even a ball-sport like water polo.

That said, if you know that you don't want to do anything other than swimming, that's okay, too! But there are still things that you can and should do within swimming to make your experience more engaging. If you feel tired of going to the pool and swimming the same sets, try some sprint workouts. If you only swim alone at 5 AM at your local gym, go to a Masters team practice one afternoon. If you can't stand the thought of getting into chlorinated water, head to the nearest river or lake and try some open water swimming.

SAFELY ADD OPEN WATER SWIMMING TO YOUR ROUTINE

As is always the case when adding a specialized training technique to your routine, find a coach or group who participate in open water swimming regularly. Your best bet is to find a triathlon club or Masters team that sponsors group swims at nearby lakes, ponds, rivers, or the ocean. If you decide to make this a regular part of your training routine, I recommend replacing one of your normal swim days with an open water day. After a few weeks, you can add your pool day back into your schedule if you like.

Which Bodies of Water are Safe?

When choosing where to swim, first be sure to pick a place where swimming is allowed. In most cases, when you see a sign prohibiting swimming it is because the water is not safe to swim in. It might be contaminated with animal feces (typically bird), or chemical runoff from streets, or have glass or metal on the bottom of shallow water.

The next thing to consider is visibility. You will rarely find open water with the same clarity as a pool, and this is often very intimidating to new swimmers. My recommendation is to progress little by little. Start by staying close to the shore in water shallow enough to allow you to stand up quickly if you get scared. As you build your confidence, you can venture further out. Make sure that there is no plant life in the water before you start swimming. Nothing freaks people out faster than having your toes tickled by algae or kelp. Interestingly, swimming in crystal clear water that is very deep can be just as scary to some newbies. I recommend that you shift your gaze to your hands, focusing on your stroke technique rather than what lies beneath.

Another thing to consider is the potential for currents. This is typically only an issue when swimming in rivers, creeks, or in the ocean. While in rivers or creeks, stay near the bank so that you can get out quickly. When swimming in a new location, always take a few strokes upstream to see how strong the current is. This will give you a sense as to how far downstream you can swim before turning around to come back to your starting point. Break up the swim into several, shorter, down and back loops, instead of going for a marathon swim. As you build your strength and confidence, go for longer distances.

Swimming in the ocean is a different beast all together. The current is variable, and the waves come in and then sweep back out. In some places you may have to contend with riptides. These are invisible streams of outflowing water that cut between two lines of incoming waves. Riptides are notoriously dangerous, causing between 50 to 100 drownings every year, according to the National Weather Service.

Here are some open water safety basics:

- Find someone to teach you how to swim in open water.
- Don't swim alone if you are swimming in unsupervised areas.
- If you are going to swim in a remote location, even if you are swimming with others, tell someone where you are going and when you expect to return.

- Buy a Runner's ID tag that you can wear on your wrist or ankle. Just in case you get in trouble and are unresponsive, you want the people who are helping you to know who you are, who they should call, and whether you have any medical conditions.

- Consider buying an inflatable swim buoy that tethers around your waist. It doesn't interfere with your stroke or slow you down. But if you find yourself in a spot of bother, you can use it to keep yourself above water until help arrives, you recover enough to swim, or you can kick your way to shore. Some people will use swim noodles like the ones that your kids play with at the pool, but these are not designed, or rated to be safety floatation devices. When you consider that a well-designed buoy retails for around $40, it is a very smart investment.

- Pay close attention to the weather. If there was a recent heavy rain, the water may be more polluted than it would be otherwise. Rivers and creeks flow faster after heavy rain. High winds increase wave heights in lakes and the ocean. There are few things scarier than being in the middle of a lake when a lightning storm rolls over you, and it only takes a few seconds to check The Weather Channel app.

Now, despite having spent the past page or so warning you about all the things that can go wrong while swimming in open water, let me finish by telling you that swimming in a lake, river, or the ocean can be a transcendent experience that I strongly encourage everyone to try. Just be safe when you do!

PART 4

SWIM PRESCRIPTION WORKOUTS

Swim Prescription Workouts

The following workouts are designed for three different levels of swimming ability.

Level I swimmers are defined as someone who has minimal swimming experience but knows how to swim each of the four strokes. So, if you can't swim all fours strokes legally (not beautifully), get some lessons under your belt first, and then use this 12-week plan.

Level II swimmers are defined as those who can swim all four strokes legally, and are currently swimming, but need a structured plan to help them progress to the next level. An intermediate swimmer should be able to complete the Intermediate 12-week training plan and then progress into the advanced training plan. This plan is also appropriate for someone who was a competitive swimmer but has been out of the water for at least a year. Start with the intermediate plan and then move on to the advanced plan.

Level III swimmers are those who have been continuously swimming for at least a year and have experience with competitive swimming, either as a swimmer solely, or in triathlon.

All three training plans are designed to progressively increase the distance and intensity of the workouts over the 12 weeks. Each plan includes three days of swimming per week. I recommend doing other activities on the non-swimming days. Cross training is always a good idea for your physical and mental health, helping you avoid getting "stale." However, if you want to swim more than three days a week, there are enough unique sets in the following training plans that you can put together your own workouts. All you have to do is keep the basic format of the workouts the same.

As you will see, each workout follows the same basic pattern:

- A warm-up set
- One or two sets that include kicking, pulling, or stroke drills
- A main set that is designed to allow for recovery, pace work, or speed work, depending on the day
- A cool down set

The default stroke is freestyle. Unless the set states otherwise, you are to swim freestyle.

We use a combination of descriptions for how you should swim each set. For the first three weeks, before the first test set (100 all out for time), you will use your rating of perceived exertion (RPE) to determine how much effort to put into each set. For these sets, I have designated how much time to rest between repetitions.

There are four other instances for when you will use these RPE zones:

1. When swimming freestyle distances less than 50 yards (or meters) or longer than 200 yards.
2. When swimming any other stroke than freestyle.
3. When doing kick or pull sets.
4. When doing stroke drill sets.

There are four RPE zones:

- Light intensity: Borg 2–3, HR 61–70%
- Moderate intensity: Borg 4–6, HR 71–80%

- High intensity: Borg 7–8, HR 81–90%
- Sprint intensity: Borg 9–10, 91–100%

After you record your 100 freestyle sprint time in week 3, you can use that to determine your paces for Freestyle sets of 50, 100, or 200 yards.

In this case, there will be three zones:

- Recovery Pace, Borg 2–3
- Base Pace, Borg 4–6
- Lactate Threshold (LT) Pace, Borg 7–8

Any intensity above LT will be a sprint set, and I will designate a certain amount of rest that you should take between repetitions.

Finally, if things are too hard or too easy, adjust them until you find your sweet spot. Do this by using your HR monitor or smart watch. That said, don't be afraid to push yourself. Now, pick a plan and let's get to work. Happy swimming!

12-WEEK PROGRAM: LEVEL I

WEEK 1

DAY 1: RECOVERY		
Warm-up	6 x 50 at Light intensity on :15 rest	300
	200 Flutter kick with fins	200/500
	6 x 50 at Light intensity on :15 rest	300/800
	[25 Finger Drag Freestyle /25 Catch-up Freestyle]	
Cooldown	200 Dolphin kick with fins at Light intensity	200/1000

DAY 2: STROKE WORK		
Warm-up	4 x 100 at Light intensity on :20 rest	400
	Do three rounds of the next two sets in a round:	600/1000
	4 x [3 x 50, then 2 x 25, repeat 3 more times]	
	3 x 50 Flutter kick with fins on :10 rest, descend 1-3	
	[Descend 1-3, #1 light, #2 moderate, #3 is fast]	
	2 x 25 fast Flutter kicking with fins on :10 rest	
Cooldown	6 x 50 at Moderate intensity on :15	300/1300
	[25 Breaststroke/25 Freestyle]	

DAY 3: SPEED WORK		
Warm-up	4 x 125 at Light intensity on :15 rest	500
	[75 Freestyle/50 Backstroke]	
	8 x 25 at Light intensity on :20 rest	200/700
	[2 x 25 of each stroke in IM order]	
	Do three rounds of the next two sets in a round:	450/1150
	4 x [3 x 25, then 1 x 75, repeat 3 more times]	
	3 x 25 descend 1-3 on :15 rest	
	[Descend 1-3, #1 easy, #2 moderate, #3 is fast]	
	75 Finger Drag Freestyle at light intensity on :30 rest	
Cooldown	200 Pull with paddles and buoy at light intensity	200/1350

WEEK 2

DAY 1: RECOVERY		
Warm-up	5 x 100 at Light intensity on :20 rest	500
	16 x 25 at Light intensity on :15 [4 of each stroke swim the drill of your choice]	400/900
Cooldown	3 x 150 at Moderate intensity on :15 rest	600/1500

DAY 2: STROKE WORK		
Warm-up	400 at Light intensity swimming [50 Breaststroke/50 Freestyle]	400
	8 x 50 at Breaststroke moderate intensity on :10 [25 drill of your choice/25 Breaststroke]	400/800
	6 x 100 at Moderate intensity swimming on :15 [50 Breaststroke/50 Freestyle]	600/1400
Cooldown	200 Breaststroke kick at light intensity	200/1600

DAY 3: SPEED WORK		
Warm-up	4 x 200 at light intensity on :20	800
	8 x 50 Pull with paddles and buoy on :10 rest [Odds are light intensity; evens are moderate intensity]	400/1200
	8 x 25 at high intensity on :40 [High intensity is between moderate and sprint]	200/1400
Cooldown	4 x 100 at light intensity on :20 [50 Backstroke/50 Freestyle]	400/1800

WEEK 3

DAY 1: RECOVERY		
Warm-up	400 at Light intensity [50 Freestyle/50 Backstroke]	400
	10 x 50 at Light intensity pull with paddles on :15 rest [Do not use a buoy during this set]	500/900
	8 x 75 IM at moderate intensity with fins on :15 rest [IM means Individual Medley] [25, Butterfly/Backstroke/Breaststroke with fins]	600/1500
Cooldown	200 Backstroke kick with fins at light intensity	200/1700

DAY 2: STROKE WORK		
Warm-up	4 x 125 at Light intensity swimming on :15 [50 Freestyle/50 Backstroke/25 Breaststroke]	500
	3 x 200 kick at Moderate intensity [#1 Flutter, #2 Dolphin, #3 Breaststroke]	600/1100
	12 x 50 at Moderate intensity on :10	600/1700
Cooldown	300 Breaststroke drill at light intensity [50 Two Kicks, One Pull/50 Breaststroke with Dolphin kick]	300/2000

DAY 3: TEST DAY		
Warm-up	8 x 50 at Light intensity on :10	400
	4 x 100 at Moderate intensity flutter kick on :15 rest [Put your fins on for this set]	400/800
	16 x 25 Descend 1-4 on :10 [#1 is easy, #2 is moderate, #3 is fast, #4 is sprint]	400/1200
	100 ALL OUT SPRINT! [Record your time to the nearest second] [Use this time to determine your paces moving forward]	100/1300
Cooldown	8 x 50 Backstroke drill at Light intensity on :20 rest [Your choice of drills]	400/1700

WEEK 4

DAY 1: RECOVERY		
Warm-up	4 x 100 at Recovery Pace [First time using the table to determine your pace]	400
	8 x 50 at Recovery Pace [Pull with paddles and buoy]	400/800
	300 Kick with fins at light intensity [100 of each stroke, take off fins for Breaststroke kick]	300/1100
Cooldown	8 x 50 at Light intensity swimming on :15 rest [25 Butterfly drill, left arm, right arm, both arms/25 Freestyle]	400/1500

DAY 2: STROKE WORK		
Warm-up	4 x 100 at Recovery Pace [First time using the table to determine your pace]	400
	8 x 50 at Recovery Pace [Pull with paddles and buoy]	400/800
	300 Kick with fins at light intensity [100 of each stroke, take off fins for Breaststroke kick]	300/1100
Cooldown	8 x 50 at Light intensity swimming on :15 rest [25 Butterfly drill, left arm, right arm, both arms/25 Freestyle]	400/1500

DAY 3: SPEED WORK		
Warm-up	4 x 200 at Recovery Pace	800
	Do three rounds of the next kick set in a round: 25 at Light intensity on :5 rest 50 at Moderate intensity on :10 rest 75 at High intensity on :15 rest [Use your fins for this set]	450/1250
	Do three rounds of the next two sets in a round: 3 x 25 ALL OUT on 1:00 rest 75 at Light intensity on 1:00 rest	450/1700
Cooldown	200 Six Kick drill with fins at light intensity	200/1900

WEEK 5

DAY 1: RECOVERY		
Warm-up	8 x 125 at Light intensity on :20 rest [2 each stroke, IM order 50 drill/75 Freestyle swim] [You pick the drills, mix them up.]	1000
	8 x 75 IM rotation at moderate intensity on :10 [#1 Butterfly/Backstroke/ Breaststroke] [#2 Backstroke/Breaststroke/Freestyle] [#3 Breaststroke/Freestyle/Butterfly] [#4 Freestyle/Butterfly/Backstroke]	600/1600
	4 x 100 Pull with paddles at Recovery Pace	400/2200
	4 x 100 Flutter kick with fins at moderate intensity on :10	400/2600
	200 at Moderate intensity [record time]	200/2800
Cooldown	200 at Light intensity [perfect stroke technique]	200/3000

DAY 2: PACE WORK		
Warm-up	3 x 200 at Light intensity on :15 [100 Freestyle/100 Backstroke]	600
	8 x 50 at Moderate intensity on :10 rest [25 Butterfly/25 Backstroke]	400/1000
	3 x 100 at Base Pace 3 x 100 at LT Pace 3 x 100 at Base Pace	900/1900
Cooldown	200 Pull with paddles, no buoy at light intensity [50 Breaststroke/50 Freestyle]	200/2100

DAY 3: SPEED WORK		
Warm-up	3 x 200 at Recovery Pace	600
	300 Kick with fins at moderate intensity	300/900

	300 Stroke drill at moderate intensity [50 1-1-2 Butterfly/50 2 kicks-1 pull Breaststroke]	300/1200
	8 x 50 on 1:30 rest [#1 ALL OUT! #2 light intensity]	400/1600
Cooldown	4 x100 at Recovery Pace	400/2000

WEEK 6

DAY 1: RECOVERY		
Warm-up	200 at Light intensity perfect stroke	200
	400 Kick, no fins at light intensity [100 of each Dolphin/Flutter/Breaststroke/Flutter]	400/600
	400 Pull with paddles and buoy at moderate intensity	400/1000
	16 x 50 Drill/swim at moderate intensity on :10 rest [5 each stroke going 25 choice drill/25 swim]	800/1800
Cooldown	6 x 100 at Recovery Pace	600/2400

DAY 2: PACE WORK		
Warm-up	4 x 125 at Light intensity on :20 rest [75 Finger Drag Freestyle/50 Freestyle]	500
	10 x 50 Pull at Base Pace with paddles, no buoy	500/1000
	4 x 200 at Base Pace [Put on your fins and move faster]	800/1800
	8 x 75 IM rotation at moderate intensity on :10 rest [Put your fins for this set]	600/2400
Cooldown	2 x 300 on 2:00 rest [#1 Fast, #2 light intensity]	600/3000

DAY 3: SPEED WORK		
Warm-up	8 x 100 at Recovery Pace	1000
	Do four rounds of the next kick set in a round: 25 at Light intensity on :5 rest 50 at Moderate intensity on :10 rest 75 at High intensity on :15 rest [Use your fins for this set]	600/1600

	Do three rounds of the next set in a round: 2 x 25 Build from easy to sprint on :15 rest 25 at Light intensity on :20 rest 2 x 25 ALL OUT on :30 rest 25 at Light intensity on :30 rest	450/2050
Cooldown	200 at Light intensity, perfect stroke	200/2250

WEEK 7

	DAY 1: RECOVERY	
Warm-up	200 at Light intensity, perfect stroke	200
	200 Kick choice, no fins at Light intensity	400/1400
	3 x 500 at Moderate intensity on 2:00 rest [Maintain a stable pace and stroke throughout]	1500/2900
Cooldown	4 x 100 at Light intensity Breaststroke on :15	400/3300

	DAY 2: PACE WORK	
Warm-up	6 x 50 at Recovery Pace	300
	6 x 50 at Base Pace	300/600
	6 x 50 at LT Pace	300/900
	6 x 100 IM at Moderate intensity with fins on :10 rest [Try to keep them all around the same time.]	600/1500
	500 Pull with paddles, no buoy, 2:00 rest [Maintain a fast, steady pace]	500/1900
	Do three rounds of the next set in a round: 150 at High intensity on :10 rest 3 x 50 at Base Pace	900/2800
Cooldown	3 x 100 Breaststroke at light intensity on 2:00 rest	300/3100

	DAY 3: SPEED WORK	
Warm-up	200 at Light intensity	200
	200 Flutter kick at moderate intensity	200/400
	200 Pull with paddles and buoy at moderate intensity	200/600
	8 x 50 at Moderate intensity Backstroke on :10 rest [25 Six-Kick Backstroke drill/25 Backstroke swimming]	400/1000
	Do four rounds of the next set in a round: 3 x 25 ALL OUT Freestyle on 1:00 rest 75 at Very light intensity on 1:00 rest	600/1600
Cooldown	4 x 100 at Light intensity, perfect Backstroke on :20 rest	400/2000

WEEK 8

DAY 1: RECOVERY		
Warm-up	6 x 100 at Recovery Pace	600
	6 x 100 IM at moderate pace with fins on :10 rest [Try to keep them all around the same time.]	600/1200
	Do six rounds of the next set in a round: 3 x 50 Pull Freestyle with paddles and buoy [#1 Recovery Pace] [#2 Base Pace] [#3 LT Pace]	900/2100
	200 at Moderate intensity [Record time, compare to the last time]	200/2300
Cooldown	3 x 200 at Base Pace	600/2900

DAY 2: PACE WORK		
Warm-up	6 x 125 at Light intensity on :20 rest [50 Breaststroke/50 Backstroke/25 Butterfly]	750
	3 x 500 at Descend 1-4 Freestyle on 2:00 rest	1500/2250
	6 x 100 at Kick with fins, no board :10 rest [Kick on your back in a streamlined position.]	600/2850
	3 x 200 Build to fast at Recovery Pace [Start easy and slowly build speed up to fast]	600/3450
Cooldown	200 Pull with paddles and buoy at light intensity	200/3650

DAY 3: TEST DAY		
Warm-up	6 x 100 at Recovery Pace	600
	16 x 50 at Base Pace [Use your fins, 25 Butterfly/25 Freestyle]	800/1400
	Do three rounds of the next set in a round: 2 x 25 Build to sprint on :20 rest 2 x 25 at Very light intensity on :20 rest	300/1700

	100 ALL OUT SPRINT! [Record your time to the nearest second]	100/1800
Cooldown	200 Backstroke Two-Arm drill at light intensity	200/2000

WEEK 9

DAY 1: RECOVERY		
Warm-up	300 at Light intensity	300
	300 Pull with paddles, no buoy at light intensity	300/600
	300 Kick choice with fins at light intensity	300/900
	6 x 100 at Base Pace	600/1500
	8 x 75 IM Rotation at moderate intensity on :15	600/2100
Cooldown	Do four rounds of the next set in a round: 2 x 50 at Recovery Pace 50 Build to fast at Recovery Pace 50 High intensity at Recovery Pace	800/2900

DAY 2: PACE WORK		
Warm-up	6 x 100 at Recovery Pace	600
	3 x 200 at Base Pace	600/1200
	6 x 100 at Base Pace	600/1800
	3 x 200 at Base Pace [Trying to go 3-5 seconds faster per 200]	600/2400
	6 x 100 at LT Pace	600/3000
Cooldown	3 x 200 at Recovery Pace	600/3600

DAY 3: TEST DAY		
Warm-up	6 x 50 at Recovery Pace	300
	8 x 75 IM on :15 rest at moderate intensity [Use your fins, 25 Butterfly/25 Backstroke/25 Breaststroke]	600/900
	300 Pull with paddles and buoy at light intensity [50 Freestyle/50 Backstroke]	300/1200
	6 x 100 ALL OUT SPRINT! On 3:00 rest [Odds are Freestyle, evens are choice stroke]	600/1800
Cooldown	6 x 50 at Recovery Pace	300/2100

WEEK 10

DAY 1: RECOVERY

Warm-up	4 x 200 at Recovery Pace with fins [50 Catch-up drill/50 swim]	800
	Do three rounds of the next set in a round: 3 x 50 Choice with fins on :10 rest 150 Swim choice stroke with fins on: 20 rest [The entire set is to be done at moderate intensity]	900/1700
	4 x 200 IM with fins at fast intensity on :30 rest	800/2500
	16 x 50 Pull with paddles at moderate intensity on :10 rest [25 Breaststroke/25 Freestyle]	800/3300
Cooldown	200 at Light intensity perfect Breaststroke	200/3500

DAY 2: PACE WORK

Warm-up	4 x 125 at Light intensity on :15 rest	500
	Do three rounds of the next set in a round: 3 x 200 at LT Pace 2 x 100 at Recovery Pace	2400/2900
	8 x 75 IM at high intensity on :10 rest [Use your fins, 25 Butterfly/25 Backstroke/25 Breaststroke]	600/3500
Cooldown	200 at Recovery Pace	200/3700

DAY 3: TEST DAY

Warm-up	300 at Light intensity	300
	300 Pull with paddles and buoy at recovery intensity	300/600
	300 Kick choice with fins at moderate intensity	300/900
	300 at Light Pace	300/1200

	12 x 50 at Recovery Pace [Odds light intensity, evens high intensity]	600/1800
	Do three rounds of the next set in a round: 2 x 50 Build to sprint at Base Pace 2 x 25 ALL OUT on :30 rest	450/2250
Cooldown	2 x 200 Kick, IM order at light intensity on :20 rest	400/2650

WEEK 11

DAY 1: RECOVERY		
Warm-up	600 at Light intensity Freestyle [100 Six-Kick drill/100 swim]	600
	6 x 100 at moderate intensity on :15 rest [50 Breaststroke/50 Backstroke]	600/1200
	10 x 50 at moderate intensity on :10 rest [25 Butterfly/25 Freestyle]	500/1700
	8 x 75 kick with fins, build to fast on :15 rest	900/2800
Cooldown	4 x 100 at Recovery Pace	400/3200

DAY 2: PACE WORK		
Warm-up	6 x 100 at Recovery Pace	600
	200 Choice kick, no fins at light intensity	200/800
	6 x 100 at Base Pace	600/1400
	200 Pull with paddles, no buoy at moderate intensity [Your choice of stroke]	200/1600
	6 x 100 at LT Pace	600/2200
Cooldown	12 x 25 Pull with paddles and buoy on :05 rest [Moderate intensity, holding the same pace throughout]	300/2500

DAY 3: TEST DAY		
Warm-up	4 x 400 at Light intensity on :30 rest [50 drill your choice of stroke/50 Freestyle swim]	1600
	Do eight rounds of the next set in a round: 2 x 25 Build to sprint on :10 rest 2 x 25 ALL OUT on :05 rest 2 x 25 easy swimming at light intensity on :20 rest	1200/2800
Cooldown	8 x 50 Pull with paddles and buoy at Base Pace	400/3200

WEEK 12

DAY 1: RECOVERY		
Warm-up	12 x 75 at light intensity on :20 rest [50 Breaststroke/25 Freestyle]	600
	4 x 200 at Base Pace	800/1400
	300 Flutter kick at moderate intensity	300/1500
	12 x 50 at moderate intensity on :20 rest [25 Breaststroke/25 Freestyle]	600/2100
	200 at moderate intensity [Record time, compare to the last two times.] [You should be getting faster]	200/2400
Cooldown	3 x 200 Breaststroke at light intensity on :20 rest	600/3000

DAY 2: PACE WORK		
Warm-up	6 x 125 at Light intensity on :20 rest [75 Catch-Up Freestyle drill/50 Freestyle swim]	750
	12 x 25 Pull with paddles and buoy on :05 rest [Moderate intensity, holding the same pace throughout]	300/1800
	Do three rounds of the next set in a round: 150 at High Intensity on :05 3 x 50 at Moderate intensity on :10 rest	900/2700
	Do three rounds of the next set in a round: 8 x 50 at LT Pace 2 x 100 at Recovery Pace	1800/4500
Cooldown	200 Pull with paddles and buoy at light intensity	200/4700

DAY 3: TEST DAY		
Warm-up	6 x 50 at Recovery Pace	300
	8 x 75 IM at moderate intensity on :10 rest [Use your fins, 25 Butterfly/25 Backstroke/25 Breaststroke]	600/900

	6 x 100 ALL OUT SPRINT! On 3:00 rest [Odds are Freestyle, evens are choice stroke]	900/2700
Cooldown	8 x 50 light intensity Backstroke drill :20	400/3100

12-WEEK PROGRAM: LEVEL II

WEEK 1

DAY 1: RECOVERY		
Warm-up	8 x 50 at Light intensity on :15 rest	400
	300 Flutter kick with fins	300/700
	10 x 50 at Light intensity on :15 rest	500/1200
	[25 Finger Drag Freestyle /25 Catch-up Freestyle]	
Cooldown	300 Dolphin kick with fins at Light intensity	300/1500

DAY 2: STROKE WORK		
Warm-up	5 x 100 at Light intensity on :20 rest	500
	Do four rounds of the next two sets in a round:	800/1300
	4 x [3 x 50, then 2 x 25, repeat 3 more times]	
	3 x 50 Flutter kick with fins on :10 rest, descend 1-3	
	[Descend 1-3, #1 light, #2 moderate, #3 Is fast]	
	2 x 25 fast Flutter kicking with fins on :10 rest	
Cooldown	12 x 50 at Moderate intensity on :15	600/1900
	[25 Breaststroke/25 Freestyle]	

DAY 3: SPEED WORK		
Warm-up	4 x 125 at Light intensity on :15 rest	500
	[75 Freestyle/50 Backstroke]	
	8 x 25 at Light intensity on :20 rest	200/700
	[2 x 25 of each stroke in IM order]	
	Do four rounds of the next two sets in a round:	600/1300
	4 x [3 x 25, then 1 x 75, repeat 3 more times]	
	3 x 25 descend 1-3 on :15 rest	
	[Descend 1-3, #1 easy, #2 moderate, #3 is fast]	
	75 Finger Drag Freestyle at light intensity on :30 rest	
Cooldown	200 Pull with paddles and buoy at light intensity	200/1500

WEEK 2

DAY 1: RECOVERY		
Warm-up	6 x 100 at Light intensity on :20 rest	600
	16 x 25 at Light intensity on :15 [4 of each stroke swim the drill of your choice]	400/1000
Cooldown	4 x 200 at Moderate intensity on :15 rest	800/1800

DAY 2: STROKE WORK		
Warm-up	600 at Light intensity swimming [50 Breaststroke/50 Freestyle]	600
	12 x 50 at Breaststroke moderate intensity on :10 [25 drill of your choice/25 Breaststroke]	600/1200
	8 x 100 at Moderate intensity swimming on :15 [50 Breaststroke/50 Freestyle]	800/2000
Cooldown	200 Breaststroke kick @ light intensity	200/2200

DAY 3: SPEED WORK		
Warm-up	4 x 200 at light intensity on :20	800
	8 x 50 Pull with paddles and buoy on :10 rest [Odds are light intensity; evens are moderate intensity]	400/1200
	8 x 25 at high intensity on :40 [High intensity is between moderate and sprint]	200/1400
Cooldown	4 x 100 at light intensity on :20 [50 Backstroke/50 Freestyle]	400/1800

WEEK 3

DAY 1: RECOVERY		
Warm-up	500 at Light intensity [50 Freestyle/50 Backstroke]	500
	12 x 50 at Light intensity pull with paddles on :15 rest [Do not use a buoy during this set]	600/1100
	8 x 75 IM at moderate intensity with fins on :15 rest [IM means Individual Medley] [25, Butterfly/Backstroke/Breaststroke with fins]	600/1700
Cooldown	300 Flutter kick with fins on your back at light intensity	300/2000

DAY 2: STROKE WORK		
Warm-up	6 x 125 at Light intensity swimming on :15 [50 Freestyle/50 Backstroke/25 Breaststroke]	750
	3 x 200 kick at Moderate intensity [#1 Flutter, #2 Dolphin, #3 Breaststroke]	600/1350
	16 x 50 at Moderate intensity on :10	800/2150
Cooldown	300 Breaststroke drill at light intensity [50 Two Kicks, One Pull/50 Breaststroke with Dolphin kick]	300/2450

DAY 3: TEST DAY		
Warm-up	8 x 50 at Light intensity on :10	400
	4 x 100 at Moderate intensity flutter kick on :15 rest [Put your fins on for this set]	400/800
	16 x 25 Descend 1-4 on :10 [#1 is easy, #2 is moderate, #3 is fast, #4 is sprint]	400/1200
	100 ALL OUT SPRINT! [Record your time to the nearest second] [Use this time to determine your paces moving forward]	100/1300
Cooldown	8 x 50 Backstroke drill at Light intensity:20[Your choice of drills]	400/1700

WEEK 4

DAY 1: RECOVERY		
Warm-up	6 x 100 at Recovery Pace [First time using the TABLE to determine your Pace]	600
	12 x 50 at Recovery Pace [Pull with paddles and buoy]	600/1200
	400 Kick with fins at light intensity [100 of each stroke, take off fins for Breaststroke kick]	400/1600
Cooldown	10 x 50 at Light intensity swimming on :15 rest [25 Butterfly drill, left arm, right arm, both arms/25 Freestyle]	500/2100

DAY 2: PACE WORK		
Warm-up	3 x 400 Descend 1-3 on 1:30 rest [#1 light, #2 moderate, #3 high]	1200
	12 x 50 Pull Breaststroke at moderate intensity on :10 rest [Use your paddles for this set, no buoy]	600/1800
	10 x 100 at Base Pace [Use the TABLE to determine your Pace]	1000/2800
Cooldown	200 at Dolphin kick [Fins with no board, work on your streamline]	200/3000

DAY 3: SPEED WORK		
Warm-up	5 x 200 at Recovery Pace	1000
	Do four rounds of the next kick set in a round: 25 at Light intensity on :5 rest 50 at Moderate intensity on :10 rest 75 at High intensity on :15 rest [Use your fins for this set]	600/1600
	Do four rounds of the next two sets in a round: 3 x 25 ALL OUT on 1:00 rest 75 at Light intensity on 1:00 rest	600/2200
Cooldown	200 Six Kick drill with fins at light intensity	200/2400

WEEK 5

DAY 1: RECOVERY		
Warm-up	8 x 125 at Light intensity on :20 rest [2 each stroke, IM order 50 drill/75 Freestyle swim] [You pick the drills, mix them up.]	1000
	8 x 75 IM rotation at moderate intensity on :10 [#1 Butterfly/Backstroke/ Breaststroke] [#2 Backstroke/Breaststroke/Freestyle] [#3 Breaststroke/Freestyle/Butterfly] [#4 Freestyle/Butterfly/Backstroke]	600/1600
	6 x 100 Pull with paddles at Recovery Pace	600/2400
	6 x 100 Flutter kick with fins at moderate intensity on :10	600/3000
	200 at Moderate intensity [record time]	200/3200
Cooldown	200 at Light intensity [perfect stroke technique]	200/3400

DAY 2: PACE WORK		
Warm-up	5 x 200 at Light intensity on :15 [100 Freestyle/100 Backstroke]	1000
	12 x 50 at Moderate intensity on :10 rest [25 Butterfly/25 Backstroke]	600/1600
	4 x 100 at Base Pace 4 x 100 at LT Pace 4 x 100 at Base Pace	1200/2800
Cooldown	200 Pull with paddles, no buoy at light intensity [50 Breaststroke/50 Freestyle]	200/3000

DAY 3: SPEED WORK		
Warm-up	3 x 200 at Recovery Pace	600
	300 Kick with fins at moderate intensity	300/900
	300 Stroke drill at moderate intensity [50 1-1-2 Butterfly/50 2 kicks-1 pull Breaststroke]	300/1200

	8 x 50 on 1:30 rest	400/1600
	[#1 ALL OUT, #2 light intensity]	
Cooldown	4 x100 at Recovery Pace	400/2000

WEEK 6

DAY 1: RECOVERY		
Warm-up	300 at Light intensity perfect stroke	300
	400 Kick, no fins at light intensity	400/700
	[100 of each Dolphin/Flutter/Breaststroke/Flutter]	
	500 Pull with paddles and buoy at moderate intensity	500/1200
	20 x 50 Drill/swim at moderate intensity on :10 rest	1000/2200
	[5 each stroke going 25 choice drill/25 swim]	
Cooldown	8 x 100 at Recovery Pace	800/3000

DAY 2: PACE WORK		
Warm-up	8 x 125 at Light intensity on :20 rest	1000
	[75 Finger Drag Freestyle/50 Freestyle]	
	16 x 50 Pull at Base Pace with paddles, no buoy	800/1800
	5 x 200 at Base Pace	1000/2800
	[Put on your fins and move faster]	
	8 x 75 IM rotation at moderate intensity on :10 rest	600/3400
	[Put your fins for this set]	
Cooldown	2 x 300 on 2:00 rest	600/4000
	[#1 Fast, #2 light intensity]	

DAY 3: SPEED WORK		
Warm-up	10 x 100 at Recovery Pace	1000
	Do six rounds of the next kick set in a round:	900/1900
	25 at Light intensity on :5 rest	
	50 at Moderate intensity on :10 rest	
	75 at High intensity on :15 rest	
	[Use your fins for this set]	

	Do four rounds of the next set in a round: 2 x 25 Build from easy to sprint on :15 rest 25 at Light intensity on :20 rest 2 x 25 ALL OUT on :30 rest 25 at Light intensity on :30 rest	600/2500
Cooldown	200 at Light intensity, perfect stroke	200/2700

WEEK 7

DAY 1: RECOVERY

Warm-up	200 at Light intensity, perfect stroke	200
	200 Kick choice, no fins at Light intensity	200/400
	4 x 500 at Moderate intensity on 2:00 rest	2000/2400
	[Maintain a sTABLE pace and stroke throughout]	
Cooldown	6 x 100 at Light intensity Breaststroke on :15	600/3000

DAY 2: PACE WORK

Warm-up	6 x 50 at Recovery Pace	300
	6 x 50 at Base Pace	300/600
	6 x 50 at LT Pace	300/900
	10 x 100 IM at Moderate intensity with fins on :10 rest	1000/1900
	[Try to keep them all around the same time.]	
	500 Pull with paddles, no buoy, 2:00 rest	500/2400
	[Maintain a fast, steady pace]	
	Do four rounds of the next set in a round:	1200/3600
	150 at High intensity on :10 rest	
	3 x 50 at Base Pace	
Cooldown	4 x 100 Breaststroke at light intensity on 2:00 rest	400/4000

DAY 3: SPEED WORK

Warm-up	400 at Light intensity	400
	400 Flutter kick at moderate intensity	400/800
	400 Pull with paddles and buoy at moderate intensity	400/1200
	12 x 50 at Moderate intensity Backstroke on :10 rest	600/1800
	[25 Six-Kick Backstroke drill/25 Backstroke swimming]	
	Do six rounds of the next set in a round: 3 x 25 ALL OUT Freestyle on 1:00 rest	900/2700
	75 at Very light intensity on 1:00 rest	
Cooldown	3 x 100 at Light intensity, perfect Backstroke on :20 rest	300/3000

WEEK 8

DAY 1: RECOVERY		
Warm-up	10 x 100 at Recovery Pace	1000
	10 x 100 IM at moderate pace with fins on :10 rest [Try to keep them all around the same time.]	1000/2000
	Do six rounds of the next set in a round: 3 x 50 Pull Freestyle with paddles and buoy [#1 Recovery Pace] [#2 Base Pace] [#3 LT Pace]	900/2900
	200 at Moderate intensity [Record time, compare to the last time]	200/3100
Cooldown	5 x 200 at Base Pace	1000/4100

DAY 2: PACE WORK		
Warm-up	8 x 125 at Light intensity on :20 rest [50 Breaststroke/50 Backstroke/25 Butterfly]	1000
	4 x 500 at Descend 1-4 Freestyle on 2:00 rest	2000/3000
	10 x 100 at Kick with fins, no board :10 rest [Kick on your back in a streamlined position.]	1000/4000
	4 x 200 Build to fast at Recovery Pace [Start easy and slowly build speed up to fast]	800/4800
Cooldown	200 Pull with paddles and buoy at light intensity	200/5000

DAY 3: TEST DAY		
Warm-up	6 x 100 at Recovery Pace	600
	16 x 50 at Base Pace [Use your fins, 25 Butterfly/25 Freestyle]	800/1400
	Do three rounds of the next set in a round: 2 x 25 Build to sprint on :20 rest 2 x 25 at Very light intensity on :20 rest	300/1700

	100 ALL OUT SPRINT! [Record your time to the nearest second]	100/1800
Cooldown	200 Backstroke Two-Arm drill at light intensity	200/2000

WEEK 9

DAY 1: RECOVERY		
Warm-up	500 at Light intensity	500
	500 Pull with paddles, no buoy at light intensity	500/1000
	500 Kick choice with fins at light intensity	500/1500
	10 x 100 at Base Pace	1000/2500
	12 x 75 IM Rotation at moderate intensity on :15	900/3400
Cooldown	Do four rounds of the next set in a round:	800/4200
	2 x 50 at Recovery Pace	
	50 Build to fast at Recovery Pace	
	50 High intensity at Recovery Pace	

DAY 2: PACE WORK		
Warm-up	10 x 100 at Recovery Pace	1000
	3 x 200 at Base Pace	600/1600
	10 x 100 at Base Pace	1000/2600
	3 x 200 at Base Pace	600/3200
	[Trying to go 3-5 seconds faster per 200]	
	10 x 100 at LT Pace	1000/4200
Cooldown	3 x 200 at Recovery Pace	600/4800

DAY 3: SPEED WORK		
Warm-up	6 x 50 at Recovery Pace	300
	8 x 75 IM on :15 rest at moderate intensity	600/900
	[Use your fins, 25 Butterfly/25 Backstroke/25 Breaststroke]	
	300 Pull with paddles and buoy at light intensity	300/1200
	[50 Freestyle/50 Backstroke]	
	6 x 100 ALL OUT SPRINT! On 3:00 rest	600/1800
	[Odds are Freestyle, evens are choice stroke]	
Cooldown	6 x 50 at Recovery Pace	300/2100

WEEK 10

DAY 1: RECOVERY		
Warm-up	5 x 200 at Recovery Pace with fins [50 Catch-up drill/50 swim]	1000
	Do four rounds of the next set in a round: 3 x 50 Choice with fins on :10 rest 150 Swim choice stroke with fins on: 20 rest [The entire set is to be done at moderate intensity]	1200/2200
	5 x 200 IM with fins at fast intensity on :30 rest	1000/3200
	20 x 50 Pull with paddles at moderate intensity on :10 rest [25 Breaststroke/25 Freestyle]	1000/4200
Cooldown	200 at Light intensity perfect Breaststroke	200/4400

DAY 2: PACE WORK		
Warm-up	8 x 125 at Light intensity on :15 rest	1000
	Do four rounds of the next set in a round: 3 x 200 at LT Pace 2 x 100 at Recovery Pace	3200/4200
	8 x 75 IM at high intensity on :10 rest [Use your fins, 25 Butterfly/25 Backstroke/25 Breaststroke]	600/4800
Cooldown	200 at Recovery Pace	200/5000

DAY 3: SPEED WORK		
Warm-up	300 at Light intensity	300
	300 Pull with paddles and buoy at recovery intensity	300/600
	300 Kick choice with fins at moderate intensity	300/900
	300 at Light Pace	300/1200
	16 x 50 at Recovery Pace	800/2000

	[Odds light intensity, evens high intensity]	600/2600
	Do four rounds of the next set in a round:	
	2 x 50 Build to sprint at Base Pace	
	2 x 25 ALL OUT on :30 rest	
Cooldown	3 x 200 Kick, IM order at light intensity on :20 rest	600/3200

WEEK 11

DAY 1: RECOVERY		
Warm-up	800 at Light intensity Freestyle [100 Six-Kick drill/100 swim]	800
	8 x 100 at moderate intensity on :15 rest [50 Breaststroke/50 Backstroke]	800/1600
	12 x 50 at moderate intensity on :10 rest [25 Butterfly/25 Freestyle]	600/2200
	12 x 75 kick with fins, build to fast on :15 rest	900/3100
Cooldown	6 x 100 at Recovery Pace	600/3700

DAY 2: PACE WORK		
Warm-up	10 x 100 at Recovery Pace	1000
	200 Choice kick, no fins at light intensity	200/1200
	10 x 100 at Base Pace	1000/2200
	200 Pull with paddles, no buoy at moderate intensity [Your choice of stroke]	200/2400
	10 x 100 at LT Pace	1000/3400
Cooldown	16 x 25 Pull with paddles and buoy on :05 rest [Moderate intensity, holding the same pace throughout]	400/3800

DAY 3: SPEED WORK		
Warm-up	4 x 400 at Light intensity on .30 rest [50 drill your choice of stroke/50 Freestyle swim]	1600
	Do eight rounds of the next set in a round: 2 x 25 Build to sprint on :10 rest 2 x 25 ALL OUT on :05 rest 2 x 25 easy swimming at light intensity on :20 rest	1200/2800
Cooldown	8 x 50 Pull with paddles and buoy at Base Pace	400/3200

WEEK 12

DAY 1: RECOVERY		
Warm-up	18 x 75 at light intensity on :20 rest [50 Breaststroke/25 Freestyle]	900
	6 x 200 at Base Pace	1200/2100
	400 Flutter kick at moderate intensity	400/2500
	16 x 50 at moderate intensity on :20 rest [25 Breaststroke/25 Freestyle]	800/3300
	200 at moderate intensity [Record time, compare to the last two times.] [You should be getting faster]	200/3500
Cooldown	3 x 200 Breaststroke at light intensity on :20 rest	600/4100

DAY 2: PACE WORK		
Warm-up	8 x 125 at Light intensity on :20 rest [75 Catch-Up Freestyle drill/50 Freestyle swim]	1000
	16 x 25 Pull with paddles and buoy on :05 rest [Moderate intensity, holding the same pace throughout]	400/1400
	Do four rounds of the next set in a round: 150 at High intensity on :05 3 x 50 at Moderate intensity on :10 rest	1200/2600
	Do four rounds of the next set in a round: 10 x 50 at LT Pace 2 x 100 at Recovery Pace	2800/5400
Cooldown	200 Pull with paddles and buoy at light intensity	200/5600

DAY 3: SPEED WORK		
Warm-up	6 x 50 at Recovery Pace	300
	8 x 75 IM at moderate intensity on :10 rest [Use your fins, 25 Butterfly/25 Backstroke/25 Breaststroke]	600/900

	6 x 100 ALL OUT SPRINT! on 3:00 rest [Odds are Freestyle, evens are choice stroke]	600/1500
Cooldown	8 x 50 at light intensity Backstroke drill :20	400/1900

12-WEEK PROGRAM: LEVEL III

WEEK 1

DAY 1: RECOVERY		
Warm-up	12 x 50 at Light intensity on :15 rest	600
	300 Flutter kick with fins	300/900
	16 x 50 at Light intensity on :15 rest	800/2100
	[25 Finger Drag Freestyle /25 Catch-up Freestyle]	
Cooldown	300 Dolphin kick with fins at Light intensity	300/2400

DAY 2: STROKE WORK		
Warm-up	8 x 100 at Light intensity on :20 rest	800
	Do five rounds of the next two sets in a round:	1000/1800
	4 x [3 x 50, then 2 x 25, repeat 3 more times]	
	3 x 50 Flutter kick with fins on :10 rest, descend 1-3	
	[Descend 1-3, #1 light, #2 moderate, #3 is fast]	
	2 x 25 fast Flutter kicking with fins on :10 rest	
Cooldown	16 x 50 at Moderate intensity on :15	800/2600
	[25 Breaststroke/25 Freestyle]	

DAY 3: SPEED WORK		
Warm-up	6 x 125 at Light intensity on :15 rest	750
	[75 Freestyle/50 Backstroke]	
	16 x 25 at Light intensity on :20 rest	400/1150
	[2 x 25 of each stroke in IM order]	
	Do four rounds of the next two sets in a round:	600/1750
	4 x [3 x 25, then 1 x 75, repeat 3 more times]	
	3 x 25 descend 1-3 on :15 rest	
	[Descend 1-3, #1 easy, #2 moderate, #3 is fast]	
	75 Finger Drag Freestyle at light intensity on :30 rest	
Cooldown	200 Pull with paddles and buoy at light intensity	200/1950

WEEK 2

DAY 1: RECOVERY		
Warm-up	8 x 100 at Light intensity on :20 rest	800
	20 x 25 at Light intensity on :15 [4 of each stroke swim the drill of your choice]	500/1300
Cooldown	5 x 200 at Moderate intensity on :15 rest	1000/2300

DAY 2: STROKE WORK		
Warm-up	800 at Light intensity swimming [50 Breaststroke/50 Freestyle]	800
	16 x 50 at Breaststroke moderate intensity on :10 [25 drill of your choice/25 Breaststroke]	800/1600
	10 x 100 at Moderate intensity swimming on :15 [50 Breaststroke/50 Freestyle]	1000/2600
Cooldown	200 Breaststroke kick at light intensity	200/2800

DAY 3: SPEED WORK		
Warm-up	5 x 200 at light intensity on :20	1000
	12 x 50 Pull with paddles and buoy on :10 rest [Odds are light intensity, evens are moderate intensity]	600/1600
	12 x 25 at high intensity on :40 [High intensity is between moderate and sprint]	300/1900
Cooldown	5 x 100 at light intensity on :20 [50 Backstroke/50 Freestyle]	500/2400

WEEK 3

DAY 1: RECOVERY		
Warm-up	500 at Light intensity [50 Freestyle/50 Backstroke]	500
	12 x 50 at Light intensity pull with paddles on :15 rest [Do not use a buoy during this set]	600/1100
	12 x 75 IM at moderate intensity with fins on :15 rest [IM means Individual Medley] [25, Butterfly/Backstroke/Breaststroke with fins]	900/2000
Cooldown	300 Flutter kick with fins on your back at light intensity	300/2300

DAY 2: STROKE WORK		
Warm-up	8 x 125 at Light intensity swimming on :15 [50 Freestyle/50 Backstroke/25 Breaststroke]	1000
	3 x 300 kick at Moderate intensity [#1 Flutter, #2 Dolphin, #3 Breaststroke]	900/1900
	20 x 50 at Moderate intensity on :10	1000/2900
Cooldown	300 Breaststroke drill at light intensity [50 Two Kicks, One Pull/50 Breaststroke with Dolphin kick]	300/3100

DAY 3: TEST DAY		
Warm-up	12 x 50 at Light intensity on :10	600
	6 x 100 at Moderate intensity flutter kick on :15 rest [Put your fins on for this set]	600/1200
	16 x 25 Descend 1-4 on :10 [#1 is easy, #2 is moderate, #3 is fast, #4 is sprint]	400/1600
	100 ALL OUT SPRINT! [Record your time to the nearest second] [Use this time to determine your paces moving forward]	100/1700
Cooldown	8 x 50 Backstroke drill at Light intensity :20 [Your choice of drills]	400/2100

WEEK 4

DAY 1: RECOVERY		
Warm-up	10 x 100 at Recovery Pace [First time using the table to determine your Pace]	1000
	12 x 50 at Recovery Pace [Pull with paddles and buoy]	600/1600
	400 Kick with fins at light intensity [100 of each stroke, take off fins for Breaststroke kick]	400/2000
Cooldown	16 x 50 at Light intensity swimming on :15 rest [25 Butterfly drill, left arm, right arm, both arms/25 Freestyle]	800/2800

DAY 2: PACE WORK		
Warm-up	3 x 500 Descend 1-3 on 1:30 rest [#1 light, #2 moderate, #3 high]	1500
	16 x 50 Pull Breaststroke at moderate intensity on :10 rest [Use your paddles for this set, no buoy]	800/2300
	10 x 100 at Base Pace [Use the table to determine your Pace]	1000/3300
Cooldown	300 at Dolphin kick [Fins with no board, work on your streamline]	300/3600

DAY 3: SPEED WORK		
Warm-up	5 x 200 at Recovery Pace	1000
	Do five rounds of the next kick set in a round: 25 at Light intensity on :5 rest 50 at Moderate intensity on :10 rest 75 at High intensity on :15 rest [Use your fins for this set]	750/1750
	Do five rounds of the next two sets in a round: 3 x 25 ALL OUT on 1:00 rest 75 at Light intensity on 1:00 rest	750/2500
Cooldown	300 Six Kick drill with fins at light intensity	300/2800

WEEK 5

DAY 1: RECOVERY		
Warm-up	8 x 125 at Light intensity on :20 rest [2 each stroke, IM order 50 drill/75 Freestyle swim] [You pick the drills, mix them up.]	1000
	12 x 75 IM rotation at moderate intensity on :10 [#1 Butterfly/Backstroke/ Breaststroke] [#2 Backstroke/Breaststroke/Freestyle] [#3 Breaststroke/Freestyle/Butterfly] [#4 Freestyle/Butterfly/Backstroke]	900/1900
	10 x 100 Pull with paddles at Recovery Pace	1000/2900
	8 x 100 Flutter kick with fins at moderate intensity on :10	800/3700
	200 at Moderate intensity [record time]	200/3900
Cooldown	200 at Light intensity [perfect stroke technique]	200/4100

DAY 2: PACE WORK		
Warm-up	5 x 200 at Light intensity on :15 [100 Freestyle/100 Backstroke]	1000
	16 x 50 at Moderate intensity on :10 rest [25 Butterfly/25 Backstroke]	800/1800
	6 x 100 at Base Pace 6 x 100 at LT Pace 6 x 100 at Base Pace	1800/3600
Cooldown	400 Pull with paddles, no buoy at light intensity [50 Breaststroke/50 Freestyle]	400/4000

DAY 3: SPEED WORK		
Warm-up	5 x 200 at Recovery Pace	1000
	400 Kick with fins at moderate intensity	400/1400
	400 Stroke drill at moderate intensity [50 1-1-2 Butterfly/50 2 kicks-1 pull Breaststroke]	400/1600

	12 x 50 on 1:30 rest [#1 ALL OUT! #2 light intensity]	600/2200
Cooldown	5 x100 at Recovery Pace	500/2700

WEEK 6

DAY 1: RECOVERY		
Warm-up	400 at Light intensity perfect stroke	400
	400 Kick, no fins at light intensity [100 of each Dolphin/Flutter/Breaststroke/Flutter]	400/800
	500 Pull with paddles and buoy at moderate intensity	500/1300
	20 x 50 Drill/swim at moderate intensity on :10 rest [5 each stroke going 25 choice drill/25 swim]	1000/2300
Cooldown	10 x 100 at Recovery Pace	1000/3000

DAY 2: PACE WORK		
Warm-up	8 x 125 at Light intensity on :20 rest [75 Finger Drag Freestyle/50 Freestyle]	1000
	16 x 50 Pull at Base Pace with paddles, no buoy	800/1800
	6 x 200 at Base Pace [Put on your fins and move faster]	1200/3000
	12 x 75 IM rotation at moderate intensity on :10 rest [Put your fins for this set]	900/3900
Cooldown	2 x 300 on 2:00 rest [#1 Fast, #2 light intensity]	600/4500

DAY 3: SPEED WORK		
Warm-up	10 x 100 at Recovery Pace	1000
	Do six rounds of the next kick set in a round: 25 at Light intensity on :05 rest 50 at Moderate intensity on :10 rest 75 at High intensity on :15 rest [Use your fins for this set]	900/1900

	Do four rounds of the next set in a round: 2 x 25 Build from easy to sprint on :15 rest 25 at Light intensity on :20 rest 2 x 25 ALL OUT on :30 rest 25 at Light intensity on :30 rest	600/2500
Cooldown	200 at Light intensity, perfect stroke	200/2700

WEEK 7

DAY 1: RECOVERY		
Warm-up	400 at Light intensity, perfect stroke	400
	400 Kick choice, no fins at Light intensity	400/800
	5 x 500 at Moderate intensity on 2:00 rest [Maintain a stable pace and stroke throughout]	2500/3300
Cooldown	6 x 100 at Light intensity Breaststroke on :15	600/3900

DAY 2: PACE WORK		
Warm-up	10 x 50 at Recovery Pace	500
	10 x 50 at Base Pace	500/1000
	10 x 50 at LT Pace	500/1500
	12 x 100 IM at Moderate intensity with fins on :10 rest [Try to keep them all around the same time.]	1200/2700
	600 Pull with paddles, no buoy, 2:00 rest [Maintain a fast, steady pace]	600/3300
	Do six rounds of the next set in a round: 150 at High intensity on :10 rest 3 x 50 at Base Pace	1800/5100
Cooldown	4 x 100 Breaststroke at light intensity on 2:00 rest	400/5500

DAY 3: SPEED WORK		
Warm-up	500 at Light intensity	500
	500 Flutter kick at moderate intensity	500/1000
	500 Pull with paddles and buoy at moderate intensity	500/1500
	12 x 50 at Moderate intensity Backstroke on :10 rest [25 Six-Kick Backstroke drill/25 Backstroke swimming]	600/2100
	Do six rounds of the next set in a round: 3 x 25 ALL OUT Freestyle on 1:00 rest 75 at Very light intensity on 1:00 rest	900/3000
Cooldown	5 x 100 at Light intensity, perfect Backstroke on :20 rest	500/3500

WEEK 8

DAY 1: RECOVERY		
Warm-up	10 x 100 at Recovery Pace	1000
	12 x 100 IM at moderate pace with fins on :10 rest [Try to keep them all around the same time.]	1200/2200
	Do six rounds of the next set in a round: 3 x 50 Pull Freestyle with paddles and buoy [#1 Recovery Pace] [#2 Base Pace] [#3 LT Pace]	900/3100
	200 at Moderate intensity [Record time, compare to the last time]	200/3300
Cooldown	5 x 200 at Base Pace	1000/4300

DAY 2: PACE WORK		
Warm-up	8 x 125 at Light intensity on :20 rest [50 Breaststroke/50 Backstroke/25 Butterfly]	1000
	4 x 600 at Descend 1-4 Freestyle on 2:00 rest	2400/3400
	10 x 100 at Kick with fins, no board :10 rest [Kick on your back in a streamlined position.]	1000/4400
	6 x 200 Build to fast at Recovery Pace [Start easy and slowly build speed up to fast]	1200/5600
Cooldown	400 Pull with paddles and buoy at light intensity	400/6000

DAY 3: TEST DAY		
Warm-up	6 x 100 at Recovery Pace	600
	16 x 50 at Base Pace [Use your fins, 25 Butterfly/25 Freestyle]	800/1400
	Do three rounds of the next set in a round: 2 x 25 Build to sprint on :20 rest 2 x 25 at Very light intensity on :20 rest	300/1700

	100 ALL OUT SPRINT! [Record your time to the nearest second]	100/1800
Cooldown	200 Backstroke Two-Arm drill at light intensity	200/2000

WEEK 9

DAY 1: RECOVERY		
Warm-up	500 at Light intensity	500
	500 Pull with paddles, no buoy at light intensity	500/1000
	500 Kick choice with fins at light intensity	500/1500
	10 x 100 at Base Pace	1000/2500
	16 x 75 IM Rotation at moderate intensity on :15	1200/3700
Cooldown	Do six rounds of the next set in a round: 2 x 50 at Recovery Pace 50 Build to fast at Recovery Pace 50 High intensity at Recovery Pace	1200/4900

DAY 2: PACE WORK		
Warm-up	10 x 100 at Recovery Pace	1000
	5 x 200 at Base Pace	1000/2000
	10 x 100 at Base Pace	1000/3000
	5 x 200 at Base Pace [Trying to go 3–5 seconds faster per 200]	1000/4000
	10 x 100 at LI Pace	1000/5000
Cooldown	5 x 200 at Recovery Pace	1000/6000

DAY 3: SPEED WORK		
Warm-up	6 x 50 at Recovery Pace	300
	8 x 75 IM on :15 rest at moderate intensity [Use your fins, 25 Butterfly/25 Backstroke/25 Breaststroke]	600/900
	300 Pull with paddles and buoy at light intensity [50 Freestyle/50 Backstroke]	300/1200
	8 x 100 ALL OUT SPRINT! On 3:00 rest [Odds are Freestyle, evens are choice stroke]	800/2000
Cooldown	6 x 50 at Recovery Pace	300/2300

WEEK 10

DAY 1: RECOVERY		
Warm-up	5 x 200 at Recovery Pace with fins [50 Catch-up drill/50 swim]	1000
	Do six rounds of the next set in a round: 3 x 50 Choice with fins on :10 rest 150 Swim choice stroke with fins on: 20 rest [The entire set is to be done at moderate intensity]	1800/2800
	8 x 200 IM with fins at fast intensity on :30 rest	1600/4400
	20 x 50 Pull with paddles at moderate intensity on :10 rest [25 Breaststroke/25 Freestyle]	1000/5400
Cooldown	200 at Light intensity perfect Breaststroke	200/5600

DAY 2: PACE WORK		
Warm-up	8 x 125 at Light intensity on :15 rest	1000
	Do four rounds of the next set in a round: 4 x 200 at LT Pace 4 x 100 at Recovery Pace	4800/5800
	12 x 75 IM at high intensity on :10 rest [Use your fins, 25 Butterfly/25 Backstroke/25 Breaststroke]	900/6700
Cooldown	300 at Recovery Pace	300/7000

DAY 3: SPEED WORK		
Warm-up	300 at Light intensity	300
	300 Pull with paddles and buoy at recovery intensity	300/600
	300 Kick choice with fins at moderate intensity	300/900
	300 at Light Pace	300/1200
	16 x 50 at Recovery Pace [Odds light intensity, evens high intensity]	800/2000

	Do four rounds of the next set in a round: 2 x 50 Build to sprint at Base Pace 2 x 25 ALL OUT on :30 rest	600/2600
Cooldown	3 x 200 Kick, IM order at light intensity on :20 rest	600/3200

WEEK 11

DAY 1: RECOVERY		
Warm-up	800 at Light intensity Freestyle [100 Six-Kick drill/100 swim]	800
	8 x 100 at moderate intensity on :15 rest [50 Breaststroke/50 Backstroke]	800/1600
	12 x 50 at moderate intensity on :10 rest [25 Butterfly/25 Freestyle]	600/2200
	12 x 75 kick with fins, build to fast on :15 rest	900/3100
Cooldown	6 x 100 at Recovery Pace	600/3700

DAY 2: PACE WORK		
Warm-up	10 x 100 at Recovery Pace	1000
	200 Choice kick, no fins at light intensity	200/1200
	10 x 100 at Base Pace	1000/2200
	200 Pull with paddles, no buoy at moderate intensity [Your choice of stroke]	200/2400
	10 x 100 at LT Pace	1000/3400
Cooldown	16 x 25 Pull with paddles and buoy on :05 rest [Moderate intensity, holding the same pace throughout]	400/3800

DAY 3: SPEED WORK		
Warm-up	5 x 400 at Light intensity on :30 rest [50 drill your choice of stroke/50 Freestyle swim]	2000
	Do eight rounds of the next set in a round: 2 x 25 Build to sprint on :10 rest 2 x 25 ALL OUT on :05 rest 2 x 25 easy swimming at light intensity on :20 rest	1200/3200
Cooldown	12 x 50 Pull with paddles and buoy at Base Pace	600/3800

WEEK 12

	DAY 1: RECOVERY	
Warm-up	18 x 75 at light intensity on :20 rest	900
	[50 Breaststroke/25 Freestyle]	
	10 x 200 at Base Pace	2000/2900
	400 Flutter kick at moderate intensity	400/3300
	20 x 50 at moderate intensity on :20 rest	1000/4300
	[25 Breaststroke/25 Freestyle]	
	200 at moderate intensity	200/4500
	[Record time, compare to the last two times.]	
	[You should be getting faster]	
Cooldown	3 x 200 Breaststroke at light intensity on :20 rest	600/5100

	DAY 2: PACE WORK	
Warm-up	8 x 125 at Light intensity on :20 rest	1000
	[75 Catch-Up Freestyle drill/50 Freestyle swim]	
	16 x 25 Pull with paddles and buoy on :05 rest	400/1400
	[Moderate intensity, holding the same pace throughout]	
	Do six rounds of the next set in a round:	1800/3200
	150 at High intensity on :05	
	3 x 50 at Moderate intensity on :10 rest	
	Do four rounds of the next set in a round:	3200/6400
	12 x 50 at LT Pace	
	2 x 100 at Recovery Pace	
Cooldown	200 Pull with paddles and buoy at light intensity	200/6600

	DAY 3: SPEED WORK	
Warm-up	10 x 50 at Recovery Pace	500
	12 x 75 IM at moderate intensity on :10 rest	900/1400
	[Use your fins, 25 Butterfly/25 Backstroke/25 Breaststroke]	

	8 x 100 ALL OUT SPRINT! On 3:00 rest [Odds are Freestyle, evens are choice stroke]	800/2200
Cooldown	12 x 50 at light intensity Backstroke drill :20	600/2800

Afterword

In the spring of 2007, I had three traumatic events occur within days of each other. First, I was diagnosed with a serious, life-threatening illness. Two days later, my engagement broke apart. A week after that, it was clear that my dissertation project hadn't worked as planned and I was going to have to start all over again if I wanted to finish my PhD. The strain was immense. I began treatments for my condition eight days after my diagnosis. The side effects were miserable. It took all my energy just to think about a new dissertation topic, and by the end of the day I was exhausted.

I fell into a deep depression. The only thing that kept me going was a single-minded urge to finish my PhD. Unfortunately, I have a bad habit of shutting people out when I get sick or injured, and I did just that, but to an even greater degree. Friends and family would call, and when I did answer, I was evasive and withdrawn. I just didn't want to burden them with what I felt were my mistakes, missteps that had put me in my current position.

But I knew I had to speak to someone, so, after finding out that my university provided free counseling services to all students, I went for several sessions. What I needed was to speak to an unbiased stranger, someone who wasn't going to tell me what I wanted to hear or play devil's advocate for the sake of it. My counselor listened and asked probing questions, but didn't offer unsolicited advice, except on one point. After hearing that I'd taken a break from swimming to focus on my dissertation, she insisted that I start exercising again. In her view, even though I was exhausted, I couldn't go from a life of regular training to nothing. At that time, running and cycling were impossible; the heat alone destroyed me. So, I went back to what I knew best: swimming.

The first few sessions were short, only a few laps of the pool. But after the first swim, I felt a sense of sleepy euphoria, and I felt compelled to stay in the water. This was partly because I didn't have the energy to climb out of the pool, but more importantly, the water was warm and welcoming. I slowly made my way underneath all the lane lines to the shallow end of the pool and squatted with the water up to my neck. I stayed perfectly still for the better part of an hour. Part of the time I had my eyes open, watching everything that was happening around me: other people swimming, the lifeguard twirling her whistle around her finger, the diving team practicing. Between those periods of quiet observation, I would close my eyes, take a deep breath, and submerge all the way underwater and sit on the pool floor. I could hear the silence of the water on my eardrums. Soon enough I could hear my heart beating. By the end of my hour of floating, I could literally hear my blood moving through my body.

I left the pool that day feeling better than I had in weeks. On my way home, my mind was clear and alert, but relaxed and calm at the same time. When I slid under the covers, I fell into a deep sleep, the likes of which I had not experienced in months. The next day I felt that something had changed. I could think again. Within a week, I had come up with a new idea for my dissertation and my appetite was slowly returning. I was not better yet, but I was on the right path. I swam every day of the week, usually early in the morning, but if an experiment ran long, I would swim at night.

After 12 weeks of treatments, I was given the all clear—I was officially in remission. I kept swimming. Over the next eight months, I started a new job as an assistant professor, wrote and defended my dissertation, and began a new life in San Antonio. I will always credit being in the water as part of my successful treatment, not just for the disease that gripped my body, but also for my soul.

I have been involved in water sports my entire life. Of all the aspects of swimming that are beneficial to our health, those related to brain health and function are the most fascinating to me. To fully measure the health outcomes of swimming, we must observe these changes through an objective, scientific lens. But it has also been my personal experience that the effects of the simple act of wading into a pool transcend scientific analysis. I can't quantify how I felt during my first, one-hour meditation session in the pool after a radiation treatment. I can only tell you that for that one hour, being in the water changed my life for the better. Although I am thankful for the scientific studies that have confirmed my feelings, in this one area, I am content with my subjective explanation, and I invite you to try it for yourself. If you're not ready to swim just yet, try jogging, walking, standing, or just floating in water for 20 minutes. Close your eyes, float, and…just be.

Acknowledgments

M y favorite TV show is *Pardon The Interruption* on ESPN. The two hosts, Mike Wilbon and Tony Kornheiser, are sports journalists, both of whom have numerous accolades for their writing. During a recent episode, Wilbon asked Kornheiser if he enjoyed writing. Tony's reply resonated with me: "I enjoy having written; writing is hard, Mike. Writing is really hard." I agree.

Next to my doctoral dissertation, this book has been the toughest writing challenge that I have undertaken. Making the process much easier were several important people in my life:

My lovely, intelligent, strong wife, and best friend Enjonli, who has been a constant supporter of all my endeavors.

My amazing daughter Kaya, who serves as a constant source of inspiration with her tenacious sporting spirit and her boundless curiosity.

My mother Julie, who read the first draft of this book cover to cover, editing all my spelling and grammatical errors.

My father James, who always serves as a sounding board for my writing ideas.

My sister Grayce and bother-in-law David, the two best siblings a big brother could ask for.

I must also thank three fellow coaches who helped me collect the data for the pace equations: Pete Covey of Alamo Area Aquatics, Tim Waud of Oregon City Tankers, and Gilberto Junior of O2 Performance Aquatics.

Finally, I must thank my friends at Hatherleigh Press who worked tirelessly during the editorial process to bring this book to fruition.

Reference Tables

50 REPEATS BASE PACE (BORG 4–6)

100 Time	Faster	Slower	Exact
0:50	0:40	0:45	0:40
0:51	0:40	0:45	0:41
0:52	0:40	0:45	0:41
0:53	0:40	0:45	0:41
0:54	0:40	0:45	0:42
0:55	0:40	0:45	0:42
0:56	0:40	0:45	0:42
0:57	0:40	0:45	0:43
0:58	0:40	0:45	0:43
0:59	0:40	0:45	0:44
1:00	0:40	0:45	0:44
1:01	0:40	0:45	0:44
1:02	0:40	0:45	0:45
1:03	0:45	0:50	0:45
1:04	0:45	0:50	0:45
1:05	0:45	0:50	0:46
1:06	0:45	0:50	0:46
1:07	0:45	0:50	0:47
1:08	0:45	0:50	0:47

50 REPEATS BASE PACE (BORG 4–6)

100 Time	Faster	Slower	Exact
1:09	0:45	0:50	0:47
1:10	0:45	0:50	0:48
1:11	0:45	0:50	0:48
1:12	0:45	0:50	0:48
1:13	0:45	0:50	0:49
1:14	0:45	0:50	0:49
1:15	0:45	0:50	0:50
1:16	0:50	0:55	0:50
1:17	0:50	0:55	0:50
1:18	0:50	0:55	0:51
1:19	0:50	0:55	0:51
1:20	0:50	0:55	0:52
1:21	0:50	0:55	0:52
1:22	0:50	0:55	0:52
1:23	0:50	0:55	0:53
1:24	0:50	0:55	0:53
1:25	0:50	0:55	0:53
1:26	0:50	0:55	0:54
1:27	0:50	0:55	0:54

50 REPEATS BASE PACE (BORG 4–6)

100 Time	Faster	Slower	Exact
1:28	0:50	0:55	0:55
1:29	0:50	0:55	0:55
1:30	0:55	1:00	0:55
1:31	0:55	1:00	0:56
1:32	0:55	1:00	0:56
1:33	0:55	1:00	0:56
1:34	0:55	1:00	0:57
1:35	0:55	1:00	0:57
1:36	0:55	1:00	0:58
1:37	0:55	1:00	0:58
1:38	0:55	1:00	0:58
1:39	0:55	1:00	0:59
1:40	0:55	1:00	0:59
1:41	0:55	1:00	1:00
1:42	0:55	1:00	1:00
1:43	1:00	1:05	1:00
1:44	1:00	1:05	1:01
1:45	1:00	1:05	1:01
1:46	1:00	1:05	1:01
1:47	1:00	1:05	1:02
1:48	1:00	1:05	1:02

50 REPEATS BASE PACE (BORG 4–6)

100 Time	Faster	Slower	Exact
1:49	1:00	1:05	1:03
1:50	1:00	1:05	1:03
1:51	1:00	1:05	1:03
1:52	1:00	1:05	1:04
1:53	1:00	1:05	1:04
1:54	1:00	1:05	1:04
1:55	1:00	1:05	1:05
1:56	1:05	1:10	1:05
1:57	1:05	1:10	1:06
1:58	1:05	1:10	1:06
1:59	1:05	1:10	1:06
2:00	1:05	1:10	1:07
2:01	1:05	1:10	1:07
2:02	1:05	1:10	1:07
2:03	1:05	1:10	1:08
2:04	1:05	1:10	1:08
2:05	1:05	1:10	1:09
2:06	1:05	1:10	1:09
2:07	1:05	1:10	1:09
2:08	1:05	1:10	1:10
2:09	1:10	1:15	1:10

50 REPEATS BASE PACE (BORG 4–6)

100 Time	Faster	Slower	Exact
2:10	1:10	1:15	1:11
2:11	1:10	1:15	1:11
2:12	1:10	1:15	1:11
2:13	1:10	1:15	1:12
2:14	1:10	1:15	1:12
2:15	1:10	1:15	1:12
2:16	1:10	1:15	1:13
2:17	1:10	1:15	1:13
2:18	1:10	1:15	1:14
2:19	1:10	1:15	1:14
2:20	1:10	1:15	1:14
2:21	1:10	1:15	1:15
2:22	1:15	1:20	1:15
2:23	1:15	1:20	1:15
2:24	1:15	1:20	1:16
2:25	1:15	1:20	1:16
2:26	1:15	1:20	1:17
2:27	1:15	1:20	1:17
2:28	1:15	1:20	1:17
2:29	1:15	1:20	1:18
2:30	1:15	1:20	1:18

50 REPEATS LT PACE (BORG 7–8)

100 Time	Faster	Slower	Exact
0:50	0:35	0:40	0:37
0:51	0:35	0:40	0:38
0:52	0:35	0:40	0:38
0:53	0:35	0:40	0:39
0:54	0:35	0:40	0:39
0:55	0:35	0:40	0:39
0:56	0:35	0:40	0:40
0:57	0:40	0:45	0:40
0:58	0:40	0:45	0:41
0:59	0:40	0:45	0:41
1:00	0:40	0:45	0:42
1:01	0:40	0:45	0:42
1:02	0:40	0:45	0:42
1:03	0:40	0:45	0:43
1:04	0:40	0:45	0:43
1:05	0:40	0:45	0:44
1:06	0:40	0:45	0:44
1:07	0:40	0:45	0:45
1:08	0:45	0:50	0:45
1:09	0:45	0:50	0:45
1:10	0:45	0:50	0:46

50 REPEATS LT PACE (BORG 7–8)

100 Time	Faster	Slower	Exact
1:11	0:45	0:50	0:46
1:12	0:45	0:50	0:47
1:13	0:45	0:50	0:47
1:14	0:45	0:50	0:48
1:15	0:45	0:50	0:48
1:16	0:45	0:50	0:48
1:17	0:45	0:50	0:49
1:18	0:45	0:50	0:49
1:19	0:45	0:50	0:50
1:20	0:50	0:55	0:50
1:21	0:50	0:55	0:51
1:22	0:50	0:55	0:51
1:23	0:50	0:55	0:51
1:24	0:50	0:55	0:52
1:25	0:50	0:55	0:52
1:26	0:50	0:55	0:53
1:27	0:50	0:55	0:53
1:28	0:50	0:55	0:54
1:29	0:50	0:55	0:54
1:30	0:50	0:55	0:54
1:31	0:50	0:55	0:55

50 REPEATS LT PACE (BORG 7–8)

100 Time	Faster	Slower	Exact
1:32	0:55	1:00	0:55
1:33	0:55	1:00	0:56
1:34	0:55	1:00	0:56
1:35	0:55	1:00	0:57
1:36	0:55	1:00	0:57
1:37	0:55	1:00	0:57
1:38	0:55	1:00	0:58
1:39	0:55	1:00	0:58
1:40	0:55	1:00	0:59
1:41	0:55	1:00	0:59
1:42	0:55	1:00	1:00
1:43	0:55	1:00	1:00
1:44	1:00	1:05	1:00
1:45	1:00	1:05	1:01
1:46	1:00	1:05	1:01
1:47	1:00	1:05	1:02
1:48	1:00	1:05	1:02
1:49	1:00	1:05	1:03
1:50	1:00	1:05	1:03
1:51	1:00	1:05	1:03
1:52	1:00	1:05	1:04

50 REPEATS LT PACE (BORG 7–8)

100 Time	Faster	Slower	Exact
1:53	1:00	1:05	1:04
1:54	1:00	1:05	1:05
1:55	1:05	1:10	1:05
1:56	1:05	1:10	1:06
1:57	1:05	1:10	1:06
1:58	1:05	1:10	1:06
1:59	1:05	1:10	1:07
2:00	1:05	1:10	1:07
2:01	1:05	1:10	1:08
2:02	1:05	1:10	1:08
2:03	1:05	1:10	1:09
2:04	1:05	1:10	1:09
2:05	1:05	1:10	1:09
2:06	1:05	1:10	1:10
2:07	1:10	1:15	1:10
2:08	1:10	1:15	1:11
2:09	1:10	1:15	1:11
2:10	1:10	1:15	1:11
2:11	1:10	1:15	1:12

50 REPEATS LT PACE (BORG 7–8)

100 Time	Faster	Slower	Exact
2:12	1:10	1:15	1:12
2:13	1:10	1:15	1:13
2:14	1:10	1:15	1:13
2:15	1:10	1:15	1:14
2:16	1:10	1:15	1:14
2:17	1:10	1:15	1:14
2:18	1:10	1:15	1:15
2:19	1:15	1:20	1:15
2:20	1:15	1:20	1:16
2:21	1:15	1:20	1:16
2:22	1:15	1:20	1:17
2:23	1:15	1:20	1:17
2:24	1:15	1:20	1:17
2:25	1:15	1:20	1:18
2:26	1:15	1:20	1:18
2:27	1:15	1:20	1:19
2:28	1:15	1:20	1:19
2:29	1:15	1:20	1:20
2:30	1:20	1:25	1:20

50 REPEATS RECOVERY PACE (BORG 2–3)

100 TIME	Faster	Slower	Exact
0:50	0:45	0:50	0:46
0:51	0:45	0:50	0:46
0:52	0:45	0:50	0:47
0:53	0:45	0:50	0:47
0:54	0:45	0:50	0:47
0:55	0:45	0:50	0:48
0:56	0:45	0:50	0:48
0:57	0:45	0:50	0:48
0:58	0:45	0:50	0:49
0:59	0:45	0:50	0:49
1:00	0:45	0:50	0:49
1:01	0:45	0:50	0:50
1:02	0:45	0:50	0:50
1:03	0:50	0:55	0:50
1:04	0:50	0:55	0:51
1:05	0:50	0:55	0:51
1:06	0:50	0:55	0:51
1:07	0:50	0:55	0:52
1:08	0:50	0:55	0:52
1:09	0:50	0:55	0:52
1:10	0:50	0:55	0:53

50 REPEATS RECOVERY PACE (BORG 2–3)

100 TIME	Faster	Slower	Exact
1:11	0:50	0:55	0:53
1:12	0:50	0:55	0:53
1:13	0:50	0:55	0:54
1:14	0:50	0:55	0:54
1:15	0:50	0:55	0:54
1:16	0:50	0:55	0:55
1:17	0:50	0:55	0:55
1:18	0:55	1:00	0:55
1:19	0:55	1:00	0:56
1:20	0:55	1:00	0:56
1:21	0:55	1:00	0:56
1:22	0:55	1:00	0:57
1:23	0:55	1:00	0:57
1:24	0:55	1:00	0:57
1:25	0:55	1:00	0:58
1:26	0:55	1:00	0:58
1:27	0:55	1:00	0:58
1:28	0:55	1:00	0:58
1:29	0:55	1:00	0:59
1:30	0:55	1:00	0:59
1:31	0:55	1:00	0:59

50 REPEATS RECOVERY PACE (BORG 2–3)

100 TIME	Faster	Slower	Exact
1:32	0:55	1:00	1:00
1:33	1:00	1:05	1:00
1:34	1:00	1:05	1:00
1:35	1:00	1:05	1:01
1:36	1:00	1:05	1:01
1:37	1:00	1:05	1:01
1:38	1:00	1:05	1:02
1:39	1:00	1:05	1:02
1:40	1:00	1:05	1:02
1:41	1:00	1:05	1:03
1:42	1:00	1:05	1:03
1:43	1:00	1:05	1:03
1:44	1:00	1:05	1:04
1:45	1:00	1:05	1:04
1:46	1:00	1:05	1:04
1:47	1:00	1:05	1:05
1:48	1:05	1:10	1:05
1:49	1:05	1:10	1:05
1:50	1:05	1:10	1:06
1:51	1:05	1:10	1:06
1:52	1:05	1:10	1:06

50 REPEATS RECOVERY PACE (BORG 2–3)

100 TIME	Faster	Slower	Exact
1:53	1:05	1:10	1:07
1:54	1:05	1:10	1:07
1:55	1:05	1:10	1:07
1:56	1:05	1:10	1:08
1:57	1:05	1:10	1:08
1:58	1:05	1:10	1:08
1:59	1:05	1:10	1:09
2:00	1:05	1:10	1:09
2:01	1:05	1:10	1:09
2:02	1:05	1:10	1:10
2:03	1:10	1:15	1:10
2:04	1:10	1:15	1:10
2:05	1:10	1:15	1:11
2:06	1:10	1:15	1:11
2:07	1:10	1:15	1:11
2:08	1:10	1:15	1:12
2:09	1:10	1:15	1:12
2:10	1:10	1:15	1:12
2:11	1:10	1:15	1:13
2:12	1:10	1:15	1:13
2:13	1:10	1:15	1:13

50 REPEATS RECOVERY PACE (BORG 2–3)

100 TIME	Faster	Slower	Exact
2:14	1:10	1:15	1:14
2:15	1:10	1:15	1:14
2:16	1:10	1:15	1:14
2:17	1:10	1:15	1:15
2:18	1:15	1:20	1:15
2:19	1:15	1:20	1:15
2:20	1:15	1:20	1:16
2:21	1:15	1:20	1:16
2:22	1:15	1:20	1:16
2:23	1:15	1:20	1:17
2:24	1:15	1:20	1:17
2:25	1:15	1:20	1:17
2:26	1:15	1:20	1:18
2:27	1:15	1:20	1:18
2:28	1:15	1:20	1:18
2:29	1:15	1:20	1:19
2:30	1:15	1:20	1:19

100 REPEATS BASE PACE (4–6)

100 Time	Faster	Slower	Exact
0:50	1:20	1:25	1:20
0:51	1:20	1:25	1:21
0:52	1:20	1:25	1:21
0:53	1:20	1:25	1:22
0:54	1:20	1:25	1:23
0:55	1:20	1:25	1:24
0:56	1:20	1:25	1:24
0:57	1:25	1:30	1:25
0:58	1:25	1:30	1:26
0:59	1:25	1:30	1:27
1:00	1:25	1:30	1:27
1:01	1:25	1:30	1:28
1:02	1:25	1:30	1:29
1:03	1:30	1:35	1:30
1:04	1:30	1:35	1:30
1:05	1:30	1:35	1:31
1:06	1:30	1:35	1:32
1:07	1:30	1:35	1:33
1:08	1:30	1:35	1:33
1:09	1:30	1:35	1:34
1:10	1:35	1:40	1:35

100 REPEATS BASE PACE (4–6)

100 Time	Faster	Slower	Exact
1:11	1:35	1:40	1:36
1:12	1:35	1:40	1:36
1:13	1:35	1:40	1:37
1:14	1:35	1:40	1:38
1:15	1:35	1:40	1:39
1:16	1:40	1:45	1:40
1:17	1:40	1:45	1:40
1:18	1:40	1:45	1:41
1:19	1:40	1:45	1:42
1:20	1:40	1:45	1:43
1:21	1:40	1:45	1:43
1:22	1:40	1:45	1:44
1:23	1:45	1:50	1:45
1:24	1:45	1:50	1:46
1:25	1:45	1:50	1:46
1:26	1:45	1:50	1:47
1:27	1:45	1:50	1:48
1:28	1:45	1:50	1:49
1:29	1:45	1:50	1:49
1:30	1:50	1:55	1:50
1:31	1:50	1:55	1:51

100 REPEATS BASE PACE (4–6)

100 Time	Faster	Slower	Exact
1:32	1:50	1:55	1:52
1:33	1:50	1:55	1:52
1:34	1:50	1:55	1:53
1:35	1:50	1:55	1:54
1:36	1:55	2:00	1:55
1:37	1:55	2:00	1:55
1:38	1:55	2:00	1:56
1:39	1:55	2:00	1:57
1:40	1:55	2:00	1:58
1:41	1:55	2:00	1:59
1:42	1:55	2:00	1:59
1:43	2:00	2:05	2:00
1:44	2:00	2:05	2:01
1:45	2:00	2:05	2:02
1:46	2:00	2:05	2:02
1:47	2:00	2:05	2:03
1:48	2:00	2:05	2:04
1:49	2:05	2:10	2:05
1:50	2:05	2:10	2:05
1:51	2:05	2:10	2:06
1:52	2:05	2:10	2:07

100 REPEATS BASE PACE (4–6)

100 Time	Faster	Slower	Exact
1:53	2:05	2:10	2:08
1:54	2:05	2:10	2:08
1:55	2:05	2:10	2:09
1:56	2:10	2:15	2:10
1:57	2:10	2:15	2:11
1:58	2:10	2:15	2:11
1:59	2:10	2:15	2:12
2:00	2:10	2:15	2:13
2:01	2:10	2:15	2:14
2:02	2:10	2:15	2:14
2:03	2:15	2:20	2:15
2:04	2:15	2:20	2:16
2:05	2:15	2:20	2:17
2:06	2:15	2:20	2:17
2:07	2:15	2:20	2:18
2:08	2:15	2:20	2:19
2:09	2:20	2:25	2:20
2:10	2:20	2:25	2:21
2:11	2:20	2:25	2:21

100 REPEATS BASE PACE (4–6)

100 Time	Faster	Slower	Exact
2:12	2:20	2:25	2:22
2:13	2:20	2:25	2:23
2:14	2:20	2:25	2:24
2:15	2:20	2:25	2:24
2:16	2:25	2:30	2:25
2:17	2:25	2:30	2:26
2:18	2:25	2:30	2:27
2:19	2:25	2:30	2:27
2:20	2:25	2:30	2:28
2:21	2:25	2:30	2:29
2:22	2:30	2:35	2:30
2:23	2:30	2:35	2:30
2:24	2:30	2:35	2:31
2:25	2:30	2:35	2:32
2:26	2:30	2:35	2:33
2:27	2:30	2:35	2:33
2:28	2:30	2:35	2:34
2:29	2:35	2:40	2:35
2:30	2:35	2:40	2:36

100 REPEATS LT PACE
(BORG 7–8)

100 Time	Faster	Slower	Exact
0:50	1:10	1:15	1:14
0:51	1:15	1:20	1:15
0:52	1:15	1:20	1:16
0:53	1:15	1:20	1:17
0:54	1:15	1:20	1:18
0:55	1:15	1:20	1:18
0:56	1:15	1:20	1:19
0:57	1:20	1:25	1:20
0:58	1:20	1:25	1:21
0:59	1:20	1:25	1:22
1:00	1:20	1:25	1:23
1:01	1:20	1:25	1:24
1:02	1:20	1:25	1:24
1:03	1:25	1:30	1:25
1:04	1:25	1:30	1:26
1:05	1:25	1:30	1:27
1:06	1:25	1:30	1:28
1:07	1:25	1:30	1:29
1:08	1:30	1:35	1:30
1:09	1:30	1:35	1:30
1:10	1:30	1:35	1:31

100 REPEATS LT PACE
(BORG 7–8)

100 Time	Faster	Slower	Exact
1:11	1:30	1:35	1:32
1:12	1:30	1:35	1:33
1:13	1:30	1:35	1:34
1:14	1:35	1:40	1:35
1:15	1:35	1:40	1:36
1:16	1:35	1:40	1:36
1:17	1:35	1:40	1:37
1:18	1:35	1:40	1:38
1:19	1:35	1:40	1:39
1:20	1:40	1:45	1:40
1:21	1:40	1:45	1:41
1:22	1:40	1:45	1:42
1:23	1:40	1:45	1:42
1:24	1:40	1:45	1:43
1:25	1:40	1:45	1:44
1:26	1:45	1:50	1:45
1:27	1:45	1:50	1:46
1:28	1:45	1:50	1:47
1:29	1:45	1:50	1:48
1:30	1:45	1:50	1:48
1:31	1:45	1:50	1:49

100 REPEATS LT PACE (BORG 7–8)

100 Time	Faster	Slower	Exact
1:32	1:50	1:55	1:50
1:33	1:50	1:55	1:51
1:34	1:50	1:55	1:52
1:35	1:50	1:55	1:53
1:36	1:50	1:55	1:53
1:37	1:50	1:55	1:54
1:38	1:55	2:00	1:55
1:39	1:55	2:00	1:56
1:40	1:55	2:00	1:57
1:41	1:55	2:00	1:58
1:42	1:55	2:00	1:59
1:43	1:55	2:00	1:59
1:44	2:00	2:05	2:00
1:45	2:00	2:05	2:01
1:46	2:00	2:05	2:02
1:47	2:00	2:05	2:03
1:48	2:00	2:05	2:04
1:49	2:05	2:10	2:05
1:50	2:05	2:10	2:05
1:51	2:05	2:10	2:06
1:52	2:05	2:10	2:07

100 REPEATS LT PACE (BORG 7–8)

100 Time	Faster	Slower	Exact
1:53	2:05	2:10	2:08
1:54	2:05	2:10	2:09
1:55	2:10	2:15	2:10
1:56	2:10	2:15	2:11
1:57	2:10	2:15	2:11
1:58	2:10	2:15	2:12
1:59	2:10	2:15	2:13
2:00	2:10	2:15	2:14
2:01	2:15	2:20	2:15
2:02	2:15	2:20	2:16
2:03	2:15	2:20	2:17
2:04	2:15	2:20	2:17
2:05	2:15	2:20	2:18
2:06	2:15	2:20	2:19
2:07	2:20	2:25	2:20
2:08	2:20	2:25	2:21
2:09	2:20	2:25	2:22
2:10	2:20	2:25	2:22
2:11	2:20	2:25	2:23
2:12	2:20	2:25	2:24
2:13	2:25	2:30	2:25

100 REPEATS LT PACE (BORG 7–8)

100 Time	Faster	Slower	Exact
2:14	2:25	2:30	2:26
2:15	2:25	2:30	2:27
2:16	2:25	2:30	2:28
2:17	2:25	2:30	2:28
2:18	2:25	2:30	2:29
2:19	2:30	2:35	2:30
2:20	2:30	2:35	2:31
2:21	2:30	2:35	2:32
2:22	2:30	2:35	2:33
2:23	2:30	2:35	2:34
2:24	2:30	2:35	2:34
2:25	2:35	2:40	2:35
2:26	2:35	2:40	2:36
2:27	2:35	2:40	2:37
2:28	2:35	2:40	2:38
2:29	2:35	2:40	2:39
2:30	2:40	2:45	2:40

100 REPEATS RECOVERY PACE (BORG 2–3)

100 Time	Faster	Slower	Exact
0:50	1:30	1:35	1:31
0:51	1:30	1:35	1:32
0:52	1:30	1:35	1:33
0:53	1:30	1:35	1:33
0:54	1:30	1:35	1:34
0:55	1:35	1:40	1:35
0:56	1:35	1:40	1:35
0:57	1:35	1:40	1:36
0:58	1:35	1:40	1:37
0:59	1:35	1:40	1:37
1:00	1:35	1:40	1:38
1:01	1:35	1:40	1:39
1:02	1:35	1:40	1:39
1:03	1:40	1:45	1:40
1:04	1:40	1:45	1:41
1:05	1:40	1:45	1:41
1:06	1:40	1:45	1:42
1:07	1:40	1:45	1:43
1:08	1:40	1:45	1:43
1:09	1:40	1:45	1:44
1:10	1:45	1:50	1:45

100 REPEATS RECOVERY PACE (BORG 2–3)

100 Time	Faster	Slower	Exact
1:11	1:45	1:50	1:45
1:12	1:45	1:50	1:46
1:13	1:45	1:50	1:47
1:14	1:45	1:50	1:47
1:15	1:45	1:50	1:48
1:16	1:45	1:50	1:49
1:17	1:45	1:50	1:49
1:18	1:50	1:55	1:50
1:19	1:50	1:55	1:51
1:20	1:50	1:55	1:51
1:21	1:50	1:55	1:52
1:22	1:50	1:55	1:53
1:23	1:50	1:55	1:53
1:24	1:50	1:55	1:54
1:25	1:50	1:55	1:55
1:26	1:55	2:00	1:55
1:27	1:55	2:00	1:56
1:28	1:55	2:00	1:56
1:29	1:55	2:00	1:57
1:30	1:55	2:00	1:58
1:31	1:55	2:00	1:58

100 REPEATS RECOVERY PACE (BORG 2–3)

100 Time	Faster	Slower	Exact
1:32	1:55	2:00	1:59
1:33	2:00	2:05	2:00
1:34	2:00	2:05	2:00
1:35	2:00	2:05	2:01
1:36	2:00	2:05	2:02
1:37	2:00	2:05	2:02
1:38	2:00	2:05	2:03
1:39	2:00	2:05	2:04
1:40	2:00	2:05	2:04
1:41	2:05	2:10	2:05
1:42	2:05	2:10	2:06
1:43	2:05	2:10	2:06
1:44	2:05	2:10	2:07
1:45	2:05	2:10	2:08
1:46	2:05	2:10	2:08
1:47	2:05	2:10	2:09
1:48	2:10	2:15	2:10
1:49	2:10	2:15	2:10
1:50	2:10	2:15	2:11
1:51	2:10	2:15	2:12
1:52	2:10	2:15	2:12

100 REPEATS RECOVERY PACE (BORG 2–3)

100 Time	Faster	Slower	Exact
1:53	2:10	2:15	2:13
1:54	2:10	2:15	2:14
1:55	2:10	2:15	2:14
1:56	2:15	2:20	2:15
1:57	2:15	2:20	2:16
1:58	2:15	2:20	2:16
1:59	2:15	2:20	2:17
2:00	2:15	2:20	2:18
2:01	2:15	2:20	2:18
2:02	2:15	2:20	2:19
2:03	2:20	2:25	2:20
2:04	2:20	2:25	2:20
2:05	2:20	2:25	2:21
2:06	2:20	2:25	2:22
2:07	2:20	2:25	2:22
2:08	2:20	2:25	2:23
2:09	2:20	2:25	2:24
2:10	2:20	2:25	2:24
2:11	2:25	2:30	2:25

100 REPEATS RECOVERY PACE (BORG 2–3)

100 Time	Faster	Slower	Exact
2:12	2:25	2:30	2:26
2:13	2:25	2:30	2:26
2:14	2:25	2:30	2:27
2:15	2:25	2:30	2:28
2:16	2:25	2:30	2:28
2:17	2:25	2:30	2:29
2:18	2:30	2:35	2:30
2:19	2:30	2:35	2:30
2:20	2:30	2:35	2:31
2:21	2:30	2:35	2:32
2:22	2:30	2:35	2:32
2:23	2:30	2:35	2:33
2:24	2:30	2:35	2:34
2:25	2:30	2:35	2:34
2:26	2:35	2:40	2:35
2:27	2:35	2:40	2:36
2:28	2:35	2:40	2:36
2:29	2:35	2:40	2:37
2:30	2:35	2:40	2:38

200 REPEATS BASE PACE (BORG 4–6)

100 Time	Faster	Slower	Exact
0:50	2:40	2:50	2:40
0:51	2:40	2:50	2:42
0:52	2:40	2:50	2:42
0:53	2:40	2:50	2:44
0:54	2:40	2:50	2:46
0:55	2:40	2:50	2:48
0:56	2:40	2:50	2:48
0:57	2:50	3:00	2:50
0:58	2:50	3:00	2:52
0:59	2:50	3:00	2:54
1:00	2:50	3:00	2:54
1:01	2:50	3:00	2:56
1:02	2:50	3:00	2:58
1:03	3:00	3:10	3:00
1:04	3:00	3:10	3:00
1:05	3:00	3:10	3:02
1:06	3:00	3:10	3:04
1:07	3:00	3:10	3:06
1:08	3:00	3:10	3:06
1:09	3:00	3:10	3:08
1:10	3:10	3:20	3:10

200 REPEATS BASE PACE (BORG 4–6)

100 Time	Faster	Slower	Exact
1:11	3:10	3:20	3:12
1:12	3:10	3:20	3:12
1:13	3:10	3:20	3:14
1:14	3:10	3:20	3:16
1:15	3:10	3:20	3:18
1:16	3:20	3:30	3:20
1:17	3:20	3:30	3:20
1:18	3:20	3:30	3:22
1:19	3:20	3:30	3:24
1:20	3:20	3:30	3:26
1:21	3:20	3:30	3:26
1:22	3:20	3:30	3:28
1:23	3:30	3:40	3:30
1:24	3:30	3:40	3:32
1:25	3:30	3:40	3:32
1:26	3:30	3:40	3:34
1:27	3:30	3:40	3:36
1:28	3:30	3:40	3:38
1:29	3:30	3:40	3:38
1:30	3:40	3:50	3:40
1:31	3:40	3:50	3:42

200 REPEATS BASE PACE (BORG 4–6)

100 Time	Faster	Slower	Exact
1:32	3:40	3:50	3:44
1:33	3:40	3:50	3:44
1:34	3:40	3:50	3:46
1:35	3:40	3:50	3:48
1:36	3:50	4:00	3:50
1:37	3:50	4:00	3:50
1:38	3:50	4:00	3:52
1:39	3:50	4:00	3:54
1:40	3:50	4:00	3:56
1:41	3:50	4:00	3:58
1:42	3:50	4:00	3:58
1:43	4:00	4:10	4:00
1:44	4:00	4:10	4:02
1:45	4:00	4:10	4:04
1:46	4:00	4:10	4:04
1:47	4:00	4:10	4:06
1:48	4:00	4:10	4:08
1:49	4:10	4:20	4:10
1:50	4:10	4:20	4:10
1:51	4:10	4:20	4:12
1:52	4:10	4:20	4:14

200 REPEATS BASE PACE (BORG 4–6)

100 Time	Faster	Slower	Exact
1:53	4:10	4:20	4:16
1:54	4:10	4:20	4:16
1:55	4:10	4:20	4:18
1:56	4:20	4:30	4:20
1:57	4:20	4:30	4:22
1:58	4:20	4:30	4:22
1:59	4:20	4:30	4:24
2:00	4:20	4:30	4:26
2:01	4:20	4:30	4:28
2:02	4:20	4:30	4:28
2:03	4:30	4:40	4:30
2:04	4:30	4:40	4:32
2:05	4:30	4:40	4:34
2:06	4:30	4:40	4:34
2:07	4:30	4:40	4:36
2:08	4:30	4:40	4:38
2:09	4:40	4:50	4:40
2:10	4:40	4:50	4:42
2:11	4:40	4:50	4:42
2:12	4:40	4:50	4:44
2:13	4:40	4:50	4:46

200 REPEATS BASE PACE (BORG 4–6)

100 Time	Faster	Slower	Exact
2:14	4:40	4:50	4:48
2:15	4:40	4:50	4:48
2:16	4:50	5:00	4:50
2:17	4:50	5:00	4:52
2:18	4:50	5:00	4:54
2:19	4:50	5:00	4:54
2:20	4:50	5:00	4:56
2:21	4:50	5:00	4:58
2:22	5:00	5:10	5:00
2:23	5:00	5:10	5:00
2:24	5:00	5:10	5:02
2:25	5:00	5:10	5:04
2:26	5:00	5:10	5:06
2:27	5:00	5:10	5:06
2:28	5:00	5:10	5:08
2:29	5:10	5:20	5:10
2:30	5:10	5:20	5:12

200 REPEATS LT PACE (BORG 7–8)

100 Time	Faster	Slower	Exact
0:50	2:20	2:30	2:28
0:51	2:30	2:40	2:30
0:52	2:30	2:40	2:32
0:53	2:30	2:40	2:34
0:54	2:30	2:40	2:36
0:55	2:30	2:40	2:36
0:56	2:30	2:40	2:38
0:57	2:40	2:50	2:40
0:58	2:40	2:50	2:42
0:59	2:40	2:50	2:44
1:00	2:40	2:50	2:46
1:01	2:40	2:50	2:48
1:02	2:40	2:50	2:48
1:03	2:50	3:00	2:50
1:04	2:50	3:00	2:52
1:05	2:50	3:00	2:54
1:06	2:50	3:00	2:56
1:07	2:50	3:00	2:58
1:08	3:00	3:10	3:00
1:09	3:00	3:10	3:00
1:10	3:00	3:10	3:02

200 REPEATS LT PACE (BORG 7–8)

100 Time	Faster	Slower	Exact
1:11	3:00	3:10	3:04
1:12	3:00	3:10	3:06
1:13	3:00	3:10	3:08
1:14	3:10	3:20	3:10
1:15	3:10	3:20	3:12
1:16	3:10	3:20	3:12
1:17	3:10	3:20	3:14
1:18	3:10	3:20	3:16
1:19	3:10	3:20	3:18
1:20	3:20	3:30	3:20
1:21	3:20	3:30	3:22
1:22	3:20	3:30	3:24
1:23	3:20	3:30	3:24
1:24	3:20	3:30	3:26
1:25	3:20	3:30	3:28
1:26	3:30	3:40	3:30
1:27	3:30	3:40	3:32
1:28	3:30	3:40	3:34
1:29	3:30	3:40	3:36
1:30	3:30	3:40	3:36
1:31	3:30	3:40	3:38

200 REPEATS LT PACE (BORG 7–8)

100 Time	Faster	Slower	Exact
1:32	3:40	3:50	3:40
1:33	3:40	3:50	3:42
1:34	3:40	3:50	3:44
1:35	3:40	3:50	3:46
1:36	3:40	3:50	3:46
1:37	3:40	3:50	3:48
1:38	3:50	4:00	3:50
1:39	3:50	4:00	3:52
1:40	3:50	4:00	3:54
1:41	3:50	4:00	3:56
1:42	3:50	4:00	3:58
1:43	3:50	4:00	3:58
1:44	4:00	4:10	4:00
1:45	4:00	4:10	4:02
1:46	4:00	4:10	4:04
1:47	4:00	4:10	4:06
1:48	4:00	4:10	4:08
1:49	4:10	4:20	4:10
1:50	4:10	4:20	4:10
1:51	4:10	4:20	4:12
1:52	4:10	4:20	4:14

200 REPEATS LT PACE (BORG 7–8)

100 Time	Faster	Slower	Exact
1:53	4:10	4:20	4:16
1:54	4:10	4:20	4:18
1:55	4:20	4:30	4:20
1:56	4:20	4:30	4:22
1:57	4:20	4:30	4:22
1:58	4:20	4:30	4:24
1:59	4:20	4:30	4:26
2:00	4:20	4:30	4:28
2:01	4:30	4:40	4:30
2:02	4:30	4:40	4:32
2:03	4:30	4:40	4:34
2:04	4:30	4:40	4:34
2:05	4:30	4:40	4:36
2:06	4:30	4:40	4:38
2:07	4:40	4:50	4:40
2:08	4:40	4:50	4:42
2:09	4:40	4:50	4:44
2:10	4:40	4:50	4:44
2:11	4:40	4:50	4:46

200 REPEATS LT PACE (BORG 7–8)

100 Time	Faster	Slower	Exact
2:12	4:40	4:50	4:48
2:13	4:50	5:00	4:50
2:14	4:50	5:00	4:52
2:15	4:50	5:00	4:54
2:16	4:50	5:00	4:56
2:17	4:50	5:00	4:56
2:18	4:50	5:00	4:58
2:19	5:00	5:10	5:00
2:20	5:00	5:10	5:02
2:21	5:00	5:10	5:04
2:22	5:00	5:10	5:06
2:23	5:00	5:10	5:08
2:24	5:00	5:10	5:08
2:25	5:10	5:20	5:10
2:26	5:10	5:20	5:12
2:27	5:10	5:20	5:14
2:28	5:10	5:20	5:16
2:29	5:10	5:20	5:18
2:30	5:20	5:30	5:20

200 REPEATS RECOVERY PACE (BORG 2–3)

100 Time	Faster	Slower	Exact
0:50	3:00	3:10	3:02
0:51	3:00	3:10	3:04
0:52	3:00	3:10	3:06
0:53	3:00	3:10	3:06
0:54	3:00	3:10	3:08
0:55	3:10	3:20	3:10
0:56	3:10	3:20	3:10
0:57	3:10	3:20	3:12
0:58	3:10	3:20	3:14
0:59	3:10	3:20	3:14
1:00	3:10	3:20	3:16
1:01	3:10	3:20	3:18
1:02	3:10	3:20	3:18
1:03	3:20	3:30	3:20
1:04	3:20	3:30	3:22
1:05	3:20	3:30	3:22
1:06	3:20	3:30	3:24
1:07	3:20	3:30	3:26
1:08	3:20	3:30	3:26
1:09	3:20	3:30	3:28
1:10	3:30	3:40	3:30

200 REPEATS RECOVERY PACE (BORG 2–3)

100 Time	Faster	Slower	Exact
1:11	3:30	3:40	3:30
1:12	3:30	3:40	3:32
1:13	3:30	3:40	3:34
1:14	3:30	3:40	3:34
1:15	3:30	3:40	3:36
1:16	3:30	3:40	3:38
1:17	3:30	3:40	3:38
1:18	3:40	3:50	3:40
1:19	3:40	3:50	3:42
1:20	3:40	3:50	3:42
1:21	3:40	3:50	3:44
1:22	3:40	3:50	3:46
1:23	3:40	3:50	3:46
1:24	3:40	3:50	3:48
1:25	3:40	3:50	3:50
1:26	3:50	4:00	3:50
1:27	3:50	4:00	3:52
1:28	3:50	4:00	3:52
1:29	3:50	4:00	3:54
1:30	3:50	4:00	3:56
1:31	3:50	4:00	3:56

200 REPEATS RECOVERY PACE (BORG 2–3)

100 Time	Faster	Slower	Exact
1:32	3:50	4:00	3:58
1:33	4:00	4:10	4:00
1:34	4:00	4:10	4:00
1:35	4:00	4:10	4:02
1:36	4:00	4:10	4:04
1:37	4:00	4:10	4:04
1:38	4:00	4:10	4:06
1:39	4:00	4:10	4:08
1:40	4:00	4:10	4:08
1:41	4:10	4:20	4:10
1:42	4:10	4:20	4:12
1:43	4:10	4:20	4:12
1:44	4:10	4:20	4:14
1:45	4:10	4:20	4:16
1:46	4:10	4:20	4:16
1:47	4:10	4:20	4:18
1:48	4:20	4:30	4:20
1:49	4:20	4:30	4:20
1:50	4:20	4:30	4:22
1:51	4:20	4:30	4:24
1:52	4:20	4:30	4:24

200 REPEATS RECOVERY PACE (BORG 2–3)

100 Time	Faster	Slower	Exact
1:53	4:20	4:30	4:26
1:54	4:20	4:30	4:28
1:55	4:20	4:30	4:28
1:56	4:30	4:40	4:30
1:57	4:30	4:40	4:32
1:58	4:30	4:40	4:32
1:59	4:30	4:40	4:34
2:00	4:30	4:40	4:36
2:01	4:30	4:40	4:36
2:02	4:30	4:40	4:38
2:03	4:40	4:50	4:40
2:04	4:40	4:50	4:40
2:05	4:40	4:50	4:42
2:06	4:40	4:50	4:44
2:07	4:40	4:50	4:44
2:08	4:40	4:50	4:46
2:09	4:40	4:50	4:48
2:10	4:40	4:50	4:48
2:11	4:50	5:00	4:50
2:12	4:50	5:00	4:52
2:13	4:50	5:00	4:52

200 REPEATS RECOVERY
PACE (BORG 2–3)

100 Time	Faster	Slower	Exact
2:14	4:50	5:00	4:54
2:15	4:50	5:00	4:56
2:16	4:50	5:00	4:56
2:17	4:50	5:00	4:58
2:18	5:00	5:10	5:00
2:19	5:00	5:10	5:00
2:20	5:00	5:10	5:02
2:21	5:00	5:10	5:04
2:22	5:00	5:10	5:04
2:23	5:00	5:10	5:06
2:24	5:00	5:10	5:08
2:25	5:00	5:10	5:08
2:26	5:10	5:20	5:10
2:27	5:10	5:20	5:12
2:28	5:10	5:20	5:12
2:29	5:10	5:20	5:14
2:30	5:10	5:20	5:16

About the Author

Alexander Hutchison, PhD, is a fitness and wellness expert in Dallas, Texas and the owner of The Athlete Company. The Senior Editor for the journal Advanced Biology, he has experience coaching swimming, water polo, triathlon, marathon, and most recently, strength and conditioning. After completing his master's degree in Kinesiology at Texas A&M University, Alexander was named the head swimming coach at Austin College. He received his doctorate in Exercise Physiology and Immunology at the University of Houston. He reviews for several journals in exercise science, nutrition, and immunology, and is an Associate Editor for the *Journal of Strength and Conditioning Research*. He is also the author of *Exercise Ain't Enough: HIIT, Honey, and the Hadza*.

References

Chapter 1

1. Roels, B., et al., *Specificity of VO2MAX and the ventilatory threshold in free swimming and cycle ergometry: comparison between triathletes and swimmers*. Br J Sports Med, 2005. 39(12): p. 965-8.

2. Holmer, I., *Oxygen uptake during swimming in man*. J Appl Physiol, 1972. 33(4): p. 502-9.

3. Laurent, M., et al., *Training-induced increase in nitric oxide metabolites in chronic heart failure and coronary artery disease: an extra benefit of water-based exercises?* Eur J Cardiovasc Prev Rehabil, 2009. 16(2): p. 215-21.

4. Chase, N.L.S., Xuemei; and Blair, Steven N., *Swimming and All-Cause Mortality Risk Compared With Running, Walking, and Sedentary Habits in Men*. International Journal of Aquatic Research and Education, 2008. 2(3).

Chapter 2

1. Mehrotra, P.K., et al., *Pulmonary functions in Indian sportsmen playing different sports*. Indian J Physiol Pharmacol, 1998. 42(3): p. 412-6.

2. Santos, M.L., et al., *Maximal respiratory pressures in healthy boys who practice swimming or indoor soccer and in healthy sedentary boys*. Physiother Theory Pract, 2012. 28(1): p. 26-31.

3. Kate, N.N., et al., *The Effect Of Short, Intermediate And Long Duration Of Swimming On Pulmonary Function Tests*. Journal of Pharmacy and Biological Sciences, 2012. 4(3): p. 18-20.

4. Eriksson, B.O., et al., *Long-term effect of previous swimtraining in girls. A 10-year follow-up of the "girl swimmers".* Acta Paediatr Scand, 1978. 67(3): p. 285-92.

5. Lomax, M., *Airway dysfunction in elite swimmers: prevalence, impact, and challenges.* Open Access J Sports Med, 2016. 7: p. 55-63.

6. Matsumoto, I., et al., *Effects of swimming training on aerobic capacity and exercise induced bronchoconstriction in children with bronchial asthma.* Thorax, 1999. 54(3): p. 196-201.

7. Varray, A.L., et al., *Individualized aerobic and high intensity training for asthmatic children in an exercise readaptation program. Is training always helpful for better adaptation to exercise?* Chest, 1991. 99(3): p. 579-86.

8. Varray, A.L., J.G. Mercier, and C.G. Prefaut, *Individualized training reduces excessive exercise hyperventilation in asthmatics.* Int J Rehabil Res, 1995. 18(4): p. 297-312.

9. Huang, S.W., et al., *The effect of swimming in asthmatic children— participants in a swimming program in the city of Baltimore.* J Asthma, 1989. 26(2): p. 117-21.

10. McNamara, R.J., et al., *Water-based exercise in COPD with physical comorbidities: a randomised controlled trial.* Eur Respir J, 2013. 41(6): p. 1284-91.

11. Edlund, L.D., et al., *Effects of a swimming program on children with cystic fibrosis.* Am J Dis Child, 1986. 140(1): p. 80-3.

Chapter 3

1. Downey, C., M. Kelly, and J.F. Quinlan, *Changing trends in the mortality rate at 1-year post hip fracture—a systematic review.* World J Orthop, 2019. 10(3): p. 166-175.

2.   Bellew, J.W. and L. Gehrig, *A comparison of bone mineral density in adolescent female swimmers, soccer players, and weight lifters*. Pediatr Phys Ther, 2006. 18(1): p. 19-22.

3.   Kanis, J.A., *Assessment of fracture risk and its application to screening for postmenopausal osteoporosis: synopsis of a WHO report. WHO Study Group*. Osteoporos Int, 1994. 4(6): p. 368-81.

4.   Charles, H.K., Chen, M.H., Spisz, T.S., Beck, T.J., Feldmesser, H.S., Magee, T.C., and B.P. Huang, *AMPDXA for Precision Bone Loss Measurements on Earth and in Space*. Johns Hopkins APL Tech. Dig, 2004. 25(3): p. 187-201.

5.   Magkos, F., Yannakoulia, M., Kavouras, S.A., and L.S. Sidossis, *The Type and Intensity of Exercise Have Independent and Additive Effects on Bone Mineral Density*. Int J Sports Med, 2007. 28: p. 773-779.

6.   Theocharidis, A., McKinlay, B.J., Vlachopolous, D., Josse, A.R., Falk, B., and P. Klentrou. *Effects of post exercise protein supplementation on markers of bone turnover in adolescent swimmers*. J. Int. Soc. Sports Nutr, 2020. 17(20): p. 1-11.

Chapter 4

1.   Fleck, S.J., *Body composition of elite American athletes*. Am J Sports Med, 1983. 11(6): p. 398-403.

2.   Flynn, M.G., et al., *Fat storage in athletes: metabolic and hormonal responses to swimming and running*. Int J Sports Med, 1990. 11(6): p. 433-40.

3.   Deligiannis, A., et al., *Plasma TSH, T3, T4 and cortisol responses to swimming at varying water temperatures*. Br J Sports Med, 1993. 27(4): p. 247-50.

4.   White, L.J.D., R. H.; Holland, E.; McCoy, S. C.; Ferguson, M. A., *Increased Caloric Intake Soon After Exercise in Cold Water*. International Journal of Sport Nutrition and Exercise Metabolism, 2005. 14: p. 38-47.

5. Horner, K.M., N.M. Byrne, and N.A. King, *Reproducibility of subjective appetite ratings and ad libitum test meal energy intake in overweight and obese males.* Appetite, 2014. 81: p. 116-22.

6. King, J.A., et al., *Individual Variation in Hunger, Energy Intake, and Ghrelin Responses to Acute Exercise.* Med Sci Sports Exerc, 2017. 49(6): p. 1219-1228.

7. Thackray, A.E., et al., *An acute bout of swimming increases post-exercise energy intake in young healthy men and women.* Appetite, 2020. 154: p. 104785.

Chapter 5

1. Kargarfard, M., et al., *Effect of aquatic exercise training on fatigue and health-related quality of life in patients with multiple sclerosis.* Arch Phys Med Rehabil, 2012. 93(10): p. 1701-8.

2. Castro-Sanchez, A.M., et al., *Hydrotherapy for the treatment of pain in people with multiple sclerosis: a randomized controlled trial.* Evid Based Complement Alternat Med, 2012. 2012: p. 473963.

3. Volpe, D., et al., *Comparing the effects of hydrotherapy and land-based therapy on balance in patients with Parkinson's disease: a randomized controlled pilot study.* Clin Rehabil, 2014. 28(12): p. 1210-7.

4. Declerck, M., et al., *Benefits and Enjoyment of a Swimming Intervention for Youth With Cerebral Palsy: An RCT Study.* Pediatr Phys Ther, 2016. 28(2): p. 162-9.

5. Lawson, L.M.L., L., *Feasibility of a Swimming Intervention to Improve Sleep Behaviors of Children With Autism Spectrum Disorder.* Therapeutic Recreation Journal, 2017. 51(2): p. 97-108.

6. Mills, W.K., N.; Orr,R.; Warburton, M.; Milne, N., *Does Hydro-therapy Impact Behaviours Related to Mental Health and Well-Being for Children with Autism Spectrum Disorder? A Randomised Crossover-Controlled Pilot Trial.* International Journal of Environmental Research and Public Health, 2020. 17.

Chapter 6

1. Mooventhan, A. and L. Nivethitha, *Scientific evidence-based effects of hydrotherapy on various systems of the body.* N Am J Med Sci, 2014. 6(5): p. 199-209.

Chapter 7

1. Valizadeh, R.A., S. H.; Saiiari, A., *The effect of eight weeks aerobic exercise in swimming pool on the mental health of men personnel of NISOC.* Procedia Social and Behavioral Sciences, 2011. 15: p. 1911-1916.

2. van Tulleken, C., et al., *Open water swimming as a treatment for major depressive disorder.* BMJ Case Rep, 2018. 2018.

3. Jonsson, K. and A. Kjellgren, *Promising effects of treatment with flotation-REST (restricted environmental stimulation technique) as an intervention for generalized anxiety disorder (GAD): a randomized controlled pilot trial.* BMC Complement Altern Med, 2016. 16: p. 108.

4. Feinstein, J.S., et al., *Examining the short-term anxiolytic and antidepressant effect of Floatation-REST.* PLoS One, 2018. 13(2): p. e0190292.

5. Sudeep, H.V. and K. Shyam Prasad, *Supplementation of green coffee bean extract in healthy overweight subjects increases lean mass/fat mass ratio: A randomized, double-blind clinical study.* SAGE Open Med, 2021. 9: p. 20503121211002590.

6.   Thomson, H., A. Kearns, and M. Petticrew, *Assessing the health impact of local amenities: a qualitative study of contrasting experiences of local swimming pool and leisure provision in two areas of Glasgow.* J Epidemiol Community Health, 2003. 57(9): p. 663-7.

7.   Carter, H.H., et al., *Cardiovascular responses to water immersion in humans: impact on cerebral perfusion.* Am J Physiol Regul Integr Comp Physiol, 2014. 306(9): p. R636-40.

8.   Parfitt, R., M.Y. Hensman, and S.J.E. Lucas, *Cerebral Blood Flow Responses to Aquatic Treadmill Exercise.* Med Sci Sports Exerc, 2017. 49(7): p. 1305-1312.

9.   Shoemaker, L.N., et al., *Swimming-related effects on cerebrovascular and cognitive function.* Physiol Rep, 2019. 7(20): p. e14247.